I0134130

KILLER BATHROOMS

Eliminate the 7 Killers Lurking in Your Home

How to inexpensively prevent serious bathroom-related injuries that kill over 20,000 older Americans and injure millions more

By: George Bentley, J.D., C.A.P.S.
Author and Safe Aging Expert

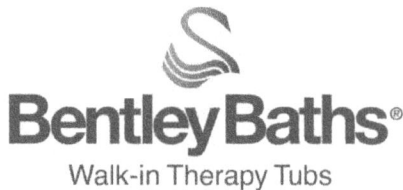

Bentley Baths®
Walk-in Therapy Tubs

www.BentleyBaths.com

Copyright, Trademark, and Disclaimer Notices

Bentley Baths®, Call Before You Fall®, Medical Hydrotherapy®, Pro-Aging™, To Bathe or Not To Bathe…That is not the Question™, and Bathe Safely…Heal Naturally™ are all registered trademarks of Bentley Wellness Technologies, Inc. and subject to the following notice

ISBN:978-0-9856213-0-8

GEORGE BENTLEY

GEORGE BENTLEY

DEDICATION

To the memory of my loving mom, who made this all happen by making the ultimate sacrifice. I am sorry we were not prepared to help you before you hurt yourself, but our experience trying to take care of you will hopefully help prevent others from going through the same fate.

To Dad, my role model as a man, my inspiration on aging with vitality and humor…no matter what. You are my "poster child" and the one who will try anything that promises to help you age better. I thank you for giving so many warm, wonderful and true stories to share with others.

GEORGE BENTLEY

What other advocates say about George's mission to help seniors:

ART LINKLETTER, lived to age 97, national chairman for the United Seniors Association, legendary radio and television host, and best-selling author of *"Old Age Is Not for Sissies"*:

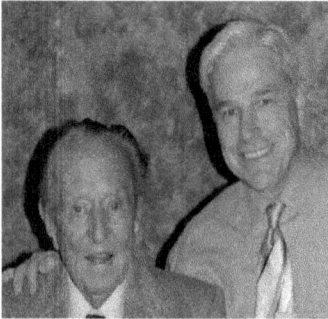

"Information is Power! George is really on a great mission to help educate and protect seniors... You should listen to George! We live between our ears. We are what we think. Your inner attitude can change the outer aspects of your life. It's real. Some people are more afraid of being old than they are of dying...The important thing is to have a positive attitude and exercise. If you don't feel safe, YOU ARE NOT SAFE. If you don't exercise, you can't feel healthy. I follow George's recommendations every day."

MARK VICTOR HANSEN, public speaker and best-selling author of the *"Chicken Soup for the Soul"* series, co-author of *"Make the Rest of Your Life the Best of Your Life"*:

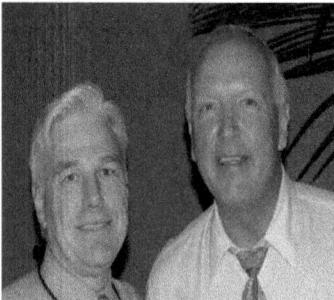

"There is such a huge need for what [George Bentley] has to offer! Our aging population is at great risk. [George] is one of those rare people who combines the knowledge and passion to offer real help to people in serious trouble... [He] has healing hands!"

KILLER BATHROOM

TABLE OF CONTENTS

GEORGE BENTLEY

ACKNOWLEDGMENTS

First, I want to thank all our amazing customers and clients, their adult children, caregivers and loved ones who have provided invaluable feedback from their experiences aging in their own homes. Katherine Bentley and Drea Knufken for their editorial review, Cassandra Heidelius for her initial organization and work, Jason Gurule for helping put it all together, and my family, for being there all the way through this process.

INTRODUCTION: A TALE OF TWO SENIORS

My parents raised my sister and me in a small town in Arkansas. We actually grew up in the house in which my mother was born. My grandmother and my grandfather both lived and, as was common in their time, died in that house.

Growing up, my mom would tell us that her intent was to do likewise. "I was born in this house, and I'm going to die in this house," she used to say. As an active kid with vastly more important things on my mind, I didn't pay much attention to her comments. But I've had good reason to remember those words later in life.

Let me explain with a "tale of two seniors." I'll set the stage for you.

Senior #1: My Mom

In 2003 my life, and the lives of my parents, took an unexpected turn. My 81-year-old mom was very healthy for her age. She worked out five times a week and I jokingly called her "Nana Schwarzenegger." Of all our relatives and friends in her generation, she was the one who was going to outlive everyone.

But one day, Mom slipped on ice as she was leaving the gym. That's right—the gym! She said she strained her leg and slightly bruised herself in that fall, but otherwise was okay. She went on about her normal routine. None of us worried too much.

A month or so later, Mom experienced a wave of lightheadedness in her bathtub. As she was trying to stand up and get out, she fell.

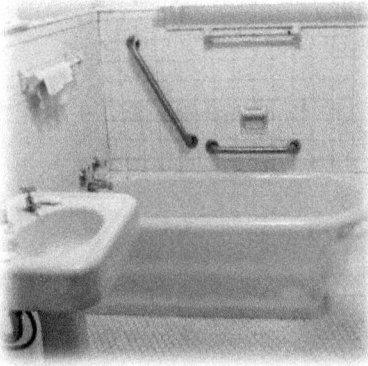

The fall really scared her, and she told my dad about it. But my parents never mentioned the bathtub fall to anyone else. Bottom line, she felt traumatized by the shock of the incident, but didn't realize she was physically injured. Although shaken, my mom didn't have any symptoms that she felt were red flags that would require diagnostic or corrective actions.

However, a day or two later, she was in "serious" pain (knowing how stoic both my parents are, I can only imagine how bad the pain had to become before she would complain). She thought it was her bowels, that the pain was being caused by a digestive tract problem (pain can be a very illusory sensation). The pain kept getting worse. She did not relate it to the bathtub incident at that point. She went over *ten days in pain,* trying to self-diagnose what was going on before finally visiting the doctor.

When she finally went to the doctor, X-rays disclosed that the fall in the bathtub had created a fracture in her pelvis (the doctor called it a stress fracture). Her injury was diagnosed as a broken hip.

This fracture was totally unknown to her after her bathtub fall. No pop, no immediate pain, just the shock of having fallen, and strain of the over-exertion as she tried to stop herself from falling out of the bathtub.

At least we now knew how she hurt herself.

After the injury is where my mom's story really starts.

My mother's bathtub injury was not serious in and of itself (a cracked pelvis, a.k.a. a broken hip). Medically speaking, she probably recovered from that injury within a few weeks.

Soon, however, she ran head-on into a very common illness I had never heard of...what's known as an "iatrogenic disease". That is, *"disease caused by receiving medical care and therapies."* That's right, we have an entire category of fatal diseases, injuries and illnesses that are caused by medications, complications, reactions, infections and other problems stemming directly from seeking medical care from a physician, pharmacist or therapist. But, I digress, that's a topic for another book.

Without the hip injury driving my mom into the hospital, it is highly possible none of the other problems would ever have occurred. Her seeking medical care set in motion a series of medical problems unrelated to the hip that caused her health to deteriorate rapidly.

First, she had a serious reaction to a pain medication. She developed what the nurses called "hospital psychosis" whereby she would rant and rave, curse and try to pull her IVs out. She was restrained with four-point restraints requiring 24/7 supervision. It really was like the *"The Exorcist"*! This was very scary to witness, especially for my father.

Mom stayed in the hospital and rehab for six weeks, due to the drug reactions, bedsores, mini-strokes and numerous other complications that evolved after the hip injury. Her cognitive abilities dropped drastically during her hospitalization.

Hospitals are not staffed to watch patients this consistently, so Dad had to hire sitters. These costs were not covered by insurance. The sitters were expensive and not all that reliable. By necessity, Dad became an employer — hiring, firing, interviewing and scheduling shifts.

How the Hospitalization and Injuries Changed Mom

When Mom finally returned home, she was not the same "Nana Schwarzenegger." She was not even "Nana" anymore. My mom was in pain, weak, disoriented and _angry!_ She had lost about 50% of her cognitive abilities. She was mean, and she vented most of her anger on my father.

Mom could no longer care for herself. My father became the primary caregiver. The physical and emotional stress he experienced dealing with Mom was palpable. In fact, my sister and I thought the stress would kill him if it continued. His quality of life was at rock bottom.

Dad fed her, helped dress her, and _tried_ his best to bathe her. This is when the bathroom once more intervened in my parent's life at home and nearly ended it all. We had no clue just how close we came to losing both our parents to this insidious _Killer Bathroom._

One time, Dad nearly dropped Mom getting her out of the tub. He injured his rotator cuff, and almost fell himself. It was only a strain, but enough to cause him to realize the danger he was putting himself in when he bathed Mom. Mom became aware that Dad was depressed, exhausted, in pain... and lonely. She realized he was physically and emotionally drained. Both my sister and I worried he would not last very long if this continued.

After staying quiet about it for a while, he finally said something to my sister and me.

The Nursing Home Spelled the End

Within nine months of her original injury in the bathroom, my dad could no longer safely help Mom bathe. Among all the other "activities of daily living" challenges he faced, bathing was *by far the worst*— and the most dangerous.

We were matter-of-factly informed by the healthcare professionals that *"your mother needs to go into a nursing home... after all, that is what they are there for."* So, we did what we thought was the right thing, put her in a nursing home.

She hated the nursing home. Every day, three times a day when he visited her, she begged my father to take her home.

Can you imagine what this was like for my dad? (Can you imagine what it was like for my mom? Well, he could, because he watched it!)

Within three months of admission into the nursing home, she was dead. We all believe she simply gave up.

Her cause of death was listed as "aspiration," meaning she choked to death on her own fluids. The real story, which was clear to those who love her, was that her fall-related injury created a direct chain of events leading straight to her death. I now know that her real cause of death was a *Killer Bathroom.*

Remember how Mom told me about her desire to die in her own home? As a child I didn't think much of it. But when I learned she had died in the nursing home, the memory from childhood came rushing back to me. When my father told me she was gone, he simply concluded: *"We failed your mother. We let her down."* I knew immediately to what he referred. My mother's words seared my memory again. I had played a role in allowing my mother to injure herself, enter a nursing home and die there, *rather than in her own home.* She died without the comfort and familiarity of the home she was born in, raised her family in, and in which she had intended to peacefully pass away.

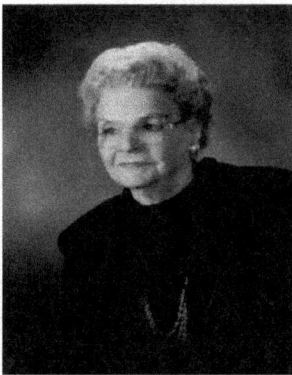

You and Dad always told me *"It's impossible to know what you don't know."* I just didn't know how to make you safer.

I am sorry, Mom.

Senior #2: My Dad

The year leading to Mom's death was obviously a very difficult one for my dad, to say the least. But, things seemed to go from bad to worse for him. His quality of life during Mom's decline was at rock bottom. He was so worried and stressed, you could feel it when he walked into the room!

Remember, Dad was depressed, exhausted, in pain ... and lonely. He was as low physically and emotionally as I had ever seen him. He even started to drink again! Both my sister and I worried he would not last very long if this continued.

It is hard for me to say, and my dad never will say, but it was actually a relief to Dad when Mom passed away. They were both suffering so much, and on some level, he realized Mom knew it!

Within two months of Mom's death, my dad was told that both his hips would need to be replaced. This development caused my dad to create another major problem in his life: *the fear of losing his independence!*

A New Death Sentence, or So He Thought

This is what the doctor said: "Mr. Bentley, I am going to replace your left hip, and you will recover from that. I will then replace your right hip, and you will recover. However, at 85, there is a small possibility that you might need a walker. You might not be able to drive, and there's a very small chance you could need a little more help getting along. You may want to move in with one of your kids or perhaps go into a nursing home. It is a good idea to be thinking ahead with your family, but you have plenty of time."

Here is what my dad heard: "Mr. Bentley, at 85 years old, after I replace your second hip, you will NOT be able to live alone. You ARE going to be forced into a nursing home to die... just like your wife!"

In his mind, my dad was being sentenced to the same fate my mom had faced — suffering alone, afraid, living his final days in a nursing home.

This, of course, traumatized my dad. My dad made it perfectly clear that he would *never* want to go into a nursing home like Mom did. He also was quite clear that he wanted to stay in his own home (my mom's family home). He was not about to move in with my family, or my sister's.

How My Dad Changed Me

My dad embodied what I have since come to respect as the strong intentions of virtually every senior and Baby Boomer I have interviewed. We, like my parents, intend to live in our own homes, and hopefully die there with as much dignity and independence as we can muster.

My dad said it plain: *"When my soul leaves this earth, I want my body going through the front door, and it is your job to help me make that happen."*

I got it.

But how could I make sure that happens? What needed to be done? When did it need to happen, and where did I find the information and resources to accomplish this objective?

I'm a lawyer, professionally trained to analyze. I'm also a visionary and a problem solver—some tease me about being "Curious George." I knew that my parents weren't unusual. This had to be happening to millions and millions of other families. And, as I am sure you know... *it is!*

I immediately began to ask questions and conduct research. "Why did this happen to my mom? What could I have done to avoid it?" I searched for the cause of the disturbing trends I found — skyrocketing hospital and nursing home admissions, an epidemic of avoidable injuries and death. An idea began to form in my head.

I thought that surely someone had thought out this problem and could tell me exactly how to help my dad. Surely someone could tell me how to prevent my dad from suffering the same fate as my mom.

Bottom line, I was informed my dad could live independently, receive in-home care, food deliveries, nursing, shuttles to the doctor's; pretty much everything he needed, that is, until he can no longer bathe safely at home. Then, he too, would be forced into a nursing home like my mother, or some other environment where he could have the support he needed.

Then the light finally went on in my head! It dawned on me that all the critical issues seemed to focus around the bathroom. The bathtub injured my mom, the bathroom and tub nearly injured my dad helping Mom, the bathtub caused Mom to go into a nursing against her will, the bathroom was now threatening my father with a similar fate.

"Curious George" Kicks into High Gear

Why is it that we can put humans in space, I can talk to my daughter in Thailand on a small plastic cell phone with no wires, we have advanced technology beyond anything our parents could ever have imagined... *and we cannot make a bathroom safe?!*

Bathtubs have remained the same basic design since the Bronze Age, over 3,300 years ago. They have been mass produced in the US since the 1880's. Yet, aside from the advent of indoor plumbing, they have remained functionally the same with no engineering modifications or accessibility design enhancements.

Then a friend told me about a Canadian company that was using a celebrity, Ed McMahon, to sell what they referred to as a "walk-in bathtub." I was on this information like white on rice. What was a "walk-in bathtub"? How did they work? Would this new technology help keep my dad at home?

I discovered that people, like my father, were being charged from $16,000 up to $20,000 (sometimes more) for one of these tubs. Man, that's expensive! But, after the initial sticker shock wore off, I had to admit, if this would keep Dad at home and safe, it was *way cheaper* than what we had been forced to pay in medical and other expenses due to Mom's fall related injuries.

I'll never forget the first time I saw one of these Premiere walk-in tubs up close. It was like a tinker toy! Cheaply built, flimsy handle, no tile flange, installed like a washing machine.

I investigated further and found that there was little to no quality control around these products, and the companies selling them were operating like the old aluminum siding sales operations of the 1960s — mass media advertising to generate leads, contract closers to high pressure the sell in the senior's living rooms (one call sales closes), followed by sub-contracted installation at the lowest possible price. Customer service and warranty were virtually non-existent.

In 2006, a widow who bought from Premiere, Phyllis Bennett, called me to say she had been sold a defective tub by this company and wanted her money back. I could not refuse to try and help her. She was an 80 year old widow, suffering from high blood pressure, chronic pain and arthritis (or the "rheumatism" as she calls it). She had previously been forced into a wheelchair following a series of back surgeries and she was living alone.

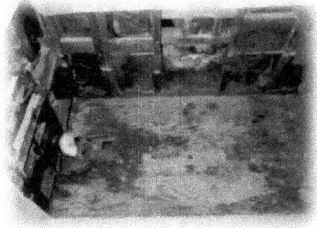

By the time she had finished pointing out all the code violations, they finally agreed to take their defective walk-in bathtub back. However, they left her with no bathtub at all! Phyllis begged me to take care of her, and help her to find a quality walk-in tub.

Thus, between helping my dad and Phyllis, I was on a new path, and a new passion in my life had been formed. It also appeared that there was a huge need in the market, and I determined that I would start a business to meet this need.

Going to every manufacturer (and there were not very many back then – most walk-in tubs were, and still are, imported), I learned about the quality, design and practical application issues that manufacturers were not focused on.

I also learned there was an advanced training program covering aging-in-place principles offered by the National Home Builder's Association, so I took the course and earned the designation of Certified Aging-in-Place Specialist.

This intensive program opened my eyes to the greater extent of the problems, and the fact that all environments pose a threat to safety as we age and manage injury or health related issues. I began conducting extensive additional research into exactly why bathrooms injure 2+ million Americans every year, and kill upwards of 20,000!

Now I have discovered the answers to many of these questions, and that is what this book is all about.

I can show you how to make your bathroom 100 times safer for under $100.

I can help you to discover *exactly* what you can do to be as safe as possible in your home for life.

Most importantly, at this writing, my dad is turning 96 years young (that's right...96!!!). He still thrives independently and lives on his own. He is living the dream that so many of us share. I wish I could have helped my mom achieve this result.

Here he is truly enjoying his beautiful "high quality walk-in bathtub with Medical Hydrotherapy®."

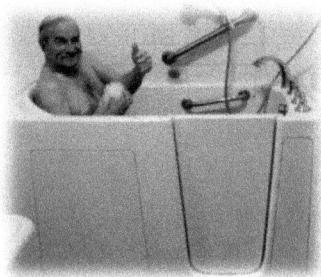

Dad, I love you, and am so grateful I was able to help you as I was not able to help Mom.

You are my "poster child"!

The Prologue

I started on a journey that has led me to not only write this book, but to research new technologies, start a business, and in short, rededicate my life.

Do other seniors, like my mom and dad, desire to live independently in their own homes? Do we know why people fall and how we can prevent these falls from ever happening? What is the cost to the families and society from these injuries? What do we do to prevent them? Are there financially or socially feasible solutions? If so, what is the best plan of action?

This book and my new passion in life are the direct result of my experience with my parents and my research.

I have become a strong proponent of what I call "Pro-Aging™" technologies, versus "anti-aging." The term "anti-aging" implies that we are "against" aging, and thus not accepting of aging as a reality.

I believe we can live happy vibrant lives in acceptance of the reality of aging. Fact is, *we all age twenty-four hours every day*. We can proactively make decisions that increase the vibrancy and quality of our lives after our 55th, or 65th, 90th, or even 100th trip around the sun.

Years of life are only one way to measure age!

We can measure our quality of life by factors such as our happiness, our vibrancy, our ability to give and contribute to others, or our medical and mental age. There is an entire body of medical science now committed to measuring our "real age" meaning the functional age of our bodies and mind without regard to the number of years we have lived.

For example, my father is medically younger at age 96 than he was when my mother died. His blood work, organ function, energy, mobility, and attitude are ALL better at 96. This is due to what he has done and the decisions he has made during those intervening years.

I believe we will see rapidly increasing numbers of Americans who easily reach 90, 100 or even more years of age with great vitality, good health and well being.

I wrote this book to help everyone avoid the *"damned if you do, damned if you don't"* dilemma that I faced.

Damned if you don't. One of the first things I learned upon starting this new journey was that I had *not* been proactive enough in helping my mother live independently in her own home. **<u>My inaction</u>** <u>contributed to my mother's death!</u>

Damned if you do. The second thing I learned was that not only did the design and engineering of the bathroom injure her, but my Band-Aid efforts to help make my mother safe actually contributed to her injury. A well meaning Occupational Therapist had told us to put a portable bench and grab bars in the tub for her. This is the "industry standard" for recommended safety modifications in the home. When Mom started to fall because the bench moved a little, she clutched at the grab bars I'd installed, and the bars' placement set her up for overexertion and the fracture. In other words... ***my actions*** *contributed to my mother's death as well!*

What I just said in the last two paragraphs is difficult for me to deal with. But it is vital information and has forever changed my outlook on aging-in-place and safety. It also led me to start questioning what some senior care professionals and therapists are recommending as "medically necessary." It is also why we came up with the tag line "Call Before You Fall®".

Knowledge is crucial, and applying solutions based on cutting-edge technologies, best practices and appreciation of the individual's unique needs can make the difference between life and death. As Dad sometimes says, "it is impossible to know what you don't know."

That is where I failed in trying to protect my mom. That is where the system failed, as well.

I lacked the knowledge to know *when to act*. This was compounded by my lack of knowledge of *how to act,* even after I'd decided to do something.

I had to come to grips with the fact that my well-meaning, uninformed efforts to help her bathe safely ended up being a primary cause of her injury in the bathroom, and therefore, her eventual death.

Finally, I realized that the cost of prevention was a drop in the bucket compared to the cost of doing nothing, *or doing the wrong thing.*

This cost, of course, does not take into account the cost of losing a loved one.

I am dedicating this book and the companion checklist to the memory of my mother. I have learned very expensive lessons from what happened to my mom.

My mother always taught me that *"Knowledge is Power!"* I hope this work will help you and your loved ones discover how to avoid making the mistakes we made with my mother's safety and care. You may also benefit from hearing about how we successfully empowered my dad to live independently in his own home, for as long as he wants... over 95 years old as of this printing, and going strong!

If I can in some small way help one person, or their loved ones, to live a safer, happier life, and achieve the goal of living independently at home for as long as possible, I know I will have made my mother proud.

THIS is the knowledge I am committed to helping you discover. This knowledge carries the power to enable you to reach that goal!

No one plans to fall and injure himself or herself! That is why we call them accidents. I want to challenge you to

DO SOMETHING TO PROTECT YOURSELF (or your parents) _BEFORE_ AN ACCIDENT HAPPENS. Once again, "Call Before You Fall®".

I also want to challenge you to learn how you can bring the truly amazing health benefits of Medical Hydrotherapy® into your home to help you overcome or delay many aging-related and degenerative health problems.

I know from my own experience, and the powerful information garnered from my research, that once the injury happens, it is often too late!

So read, learn, and then call for help! And remember, I am not suggesting that I know all there is to know. But I have learned a lot.

My commitment is to do anything I reasonably can to help you and your family, and I would be honored to have my professional staff speak with you or conduct a comprehensive safety assessment at no charge.

You have a friend and an advocate to help your family learn about specific products and technologies, so you can determine the best course of action for you! I hope you find this information helpful.

CHAPTER ONE
THE RESEARCH

TWO SILENT EPIDEMICS THREATEN OUR FUTURE:

IGNORANCE AND DENIAL

> "When I met George I politely listened to him, but told him my 89 y/o dad was 'doing ok'. A few weeks later he fell in his bathroom and broke his shoulder. Nine months later we were burying him. I wish I would have acted when I first met George. My ignorance may have contributed to his death."
>
> *Harry Lay*

One in every three adults age 65 and older falls each year. Falls can lead to moderate injuries, such as bruises, sprains and strains, or more serious injuries such as hip fractures (my mom), broken bones (Harry's dad) and head traumas. Every one of these injuries will increase the risk of early death (such as the series of iatrogenic conditions that led to my mother's death).

The Centers for Disease Control (CDC) casually states: "... fortunately, falls are a public health problem that is largely preventable." Easier said than done! Especially if we are not aware of the problem and are not knowledgeable about how to prevent the injuries! Just ask me, or Harry Lay, or any one of the millions of others who have experienced the trauma of a fall-related injury to a loved one.

As I said earlier, my company has trademarked the tagline "Call Before You Fall®" due to the very high incidence of people not realizing how great their risk of injury actually is.

Something has to happen for people to pay attention to the real risk. Right now, prevention is not a critical part of the process for safe aging in America, and at that point a fall and related injury occurs, it is often too late, like it was with my mom.

Exactly how big is the problem?

The CDC is the authoritative source for accident and health information. These statistics are taken straight from their report.

- One out of three adults age 65 and older falls each year. That's over 20 million a year! And that will steadily increase to over 26 million a year as the baby boomers age!
- Among those age 65 and older, falls are the leading cause of injury or death. They are also the most common cause of nonfatal injuries and hospital admissions for trauma.
- *In 2007, over 18,000 older adults died from*

unintentional fall injuries. That rose to 20,000 in 2009, and the number is well over that now.

- The death rate from falls among older men and women has risen sharply over the past decade, and is projected to continue to increase with the aging population.
- In 2000, direct medical costs of falls totaled over $19 billion. Based on today's population, that's over <u>$26 *billion every year*</u>!!

Here is the CDC statistic that really stopped me in my tracks:

- **In 2009, 2.2 million nonfatal fall *injuries* among older adults were treated in emergency departments and more than 581,000 of these patients were hospitalized.**

In other words, there were 2.2 million people just like my mom in 2009.

Once I'd seen these figures, I just did some simple math. And, I'll bet you have probably heard somebody somewhere cite my numbers, because once I did the math and started putting these figures in my articles, website, videos, and in the media, many others have cited my calculations to make the point.

The lowest common denominator sometimes can be the most powerful.

So, here we go.

2.2 million *medically treated* fall-related injuries per year (we are not even talking about the millions of other falls and injuries that are not formally treated by a doctor). Keep in mind that to be counted, the injury must be reported, and to be reported requires formal medical treatment. So, many falls are never reported, and are NOT part of this number.

Okay, so 2.2 million injuries a year divided by 365 days means 6,027 fall related injuries requiring formal medical treatment *every day*. Wow, 6,027 fall related injuries *a day* sounds a little more compelling. But let's go deeper.

If we take 6,027 per day divided by 24 hours this equals *over 251 fall related injuries per hour*, 24 hours a day, 7 days a week, 365 days a year! So, during the time of your lunch break every day, 251 seniors fall and hurt themselves so severely they are treated in hospitals due to their injuries.

Taking the calculation a step further, seniors are falling and injuring themselves at the rate of 251 per hour divided by 60 minutes means *4 falls per minute*.

But, for whatever reason, the next level is the number that really hits home with people. It is the data I hear picked up and used by others more often than any other statistic I have come up with to date.

Four fall-related injuries per minute means **_once every 15 seconds_**, someone's mother or father, brother or sister, aunt or uncle, friend or loved one over the age of 65 *falls and injures themselves so severely it sends them to the hospital!*

More people seem to realize just how serious this problem really is when they can hear it stated like this... "Once every 15 seconds!"

Now we've become painfully aware of the fact that many, many people are suffering and shortening their lives because of the unsafe conditions that we find in our bathrooms. The real question is: why is this happening? Why are we not doing things to make our seniors and ourselves safe?

The answer is really a combination of two converging problems. These two conditions are coming together to create "the perfect storm" of death and injury to seniors and all Americans who are dealing with age, health, weight, or injury related mobility issues.

EPIDEMIC #1:   IGNORANCE
It's Impossible to Know What You Don't Know

As I was growing up, my father was fond of reminding me that it's impossible to know what you don't know. He would frequently say this to me in situations where I was struggling to figure out an answer to a problem when I didn't have all the necessary information. This is a very appropriate analogy as it relates to seniors dealing with their bathrooms. It also very pointedly explains what happened to my family and specifically to my mother.

Who goes into their bathroom and expects *the bathroom* to change as they age? Nobody.

As I pointed out earlier, the fact remains that every day we live, every trip we take around the sun, we get a year older, we get weaker, and we become less stable. Our connective tissues weaken, our skin thins, we begin to lose our vision, and we begin to lose our hearing. These are all just facts of life. However, it is not a fact of our life to expect our bathrooms to change to accommodate us as we go through these physical changes due to age.

I have interviewed thousands of seniors, their adult children, and their caregivers, and in many of those interviews I will request that the senior demonstrate for me how they enter and exit their existing bathtub or shower. If it's at all possible, I try to arrange the situation so that the spouse, adult child or caregiver can observe this process from the bathroom door or hallway.

> "Information is Power! We live between our ears. Some people are more afraid of being old than they are of dying... If you don't feel safe, YOU ARE NOT SAFE."
>
> Art Linkletter

I now have videos of many of these transitions on the internet. Visit Bentley Baths' YouTube Channel (http://www.youtube.com/user/BentleyBaths?feature= watch) or search for "Bentley Baths" or "Senior Falls" on YouTube. Also visit our Facebook page and Blog (www.BentleyBaths.com/blog). These videos are candid and shockingly real, and are almost always the first time a spouse, adult child or loved one sees the reality of what getting into or out of a bathtub or shower can be like. I will be putting more such info up all the time, so keep checking back.

So, let's discuss what the results of my interviews revealed.

It is not uncommon for me to watch a senior struggle to analyze, with much stress and difficulty, how they're going to enter that bathtub. Many will stand outside the tub at the wall in the bathroom opposite where the valves are, face away from the valves, lean both hands against the wall to brace themselves, and then start the painful process of trying to lift first one leg, then the other, over and into the bathtub in order to transition in.

Many can't even begin to lift their leg to make this process. Those who do accomplish getting into the tub using this method are now facing the wrong direction in the tub and standing up, rather than sitting. We then watch them slowly turn themselves around, orient themselves in the tub, and then begin the process of lowering themselves onto the floor so that they can bathe. (See the video of Mr. Diass on the Bentley Baths YouTube Channel.) Scary to watch.

It's also not uncommon for me to look at a spouse or an adult child at this point and inquire: "Are you seeing this? Can you see how dangerous this process is for your wife, mom or dad?" Fact is, getting into the bathtub or shower will be one of the most dangerous things a senior will go through on any given day, week, or month. Fact is, with the inclusion of going up or down stairs, nothing is more dangerous.

Others can't even begin the process of trying to step into the tub. They will sometimes lie on the floor on all fours and attempt to throw one arm and one leg over into the tub and slide over the top edge of the bathtub in order to get into the bath itself. Once in the tub, they are, once again, usually facing the wrong direction. They have to go through the very stressful, strenuous process of trying to move their legs under their body, and turn themselves around to get situated in the bathtub.

Observing this process first hand in 100s of homes led me to conclude that "millions of seniors are suffering quietly in the bathroom!" This is exactly what my mom went through. I now understand how millions and millions of seniors are forced to determine for themselves how it is that they are going to attempt to get their aged, weak, unstable bodies into (and hopefully out of) that bathtub.

The process of entering a bathtub or shower becomes very, very difficult and many people are unwilling to acknowledge and accept this. But the obvious issue is that once I am in a bathing environment that is designed for me to lie on the floor in order to take a bath, it is only a matter of time until I will not be able to get myself back up off the floor and out of that bathtub.

That is exactly how many of the people I interviewed injured themselves. They were able to get themselves into the tub, and were able to get down on the floor to take their bath. However, after finishing the bath, they required great exertion and use of all their strength to try to get themselves up. In this wet slick environment, they slip or lose their balance, thus falling out of (or into) the bathtub.

Think the Shower is Safer? Think Again.

One thing that I encounter in my conversations with seniors is that many believe that showers are actually safer. Men in particular tend to suggest that because they often shower instead of bathing, and that by doing so they are somehow perfectly safe.

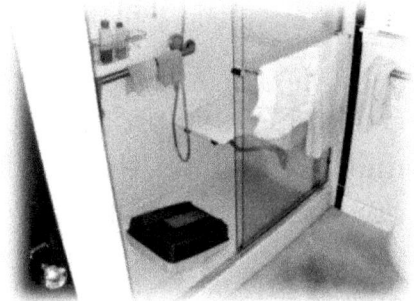

I wish that were true! But it's not. Showers, even if they have low barriers, are actually more dangerous than bathtubs. Yes, it may be somewhat easier to get my feet over the threshold of a three, four or five-inch shower pan than it is an eighteen, twenty or thirty-inch-high bathtub sidewall. Showers are designed and engineered in such a way that the bather must stand while they wash themselves. This requires that you have sufficient stability and balance so as to easily reach all your body parts from a standing position. Inserting a stool or bench into the shower means not having to stand, but the lack of stability is unchanged. Now both the person *and* the stool are unstable.

One becomes more vulnerable to fall-related injuries when moving in and out of a shower. Wet surfaces, hard surfaces, glass shower doors, moveable shower curtains, standing and moving, light-headedness or dizziness, are all factors that lead to a situation where showers are more dangerous than bathtubs. I refer to this as doing the "rain dance." It is simply NOT safe!

We are standing, unsupported and transitioning in or out in an environment that is unforgiving. The mere fact we are in a standing position means our fall related injury risk is exponentially greater than when we are seated.

The issue with bathtubs is getting into and out of them. That's dangerous, but at least while you're lying in the tub you're stable. In a shower, you are unstable and at risk throughout that entire process.

So why do we do this? Why do we go through all these gyrations and put ourselves at such risk?

Speaking for my family, we simply did not know that there were resources available to help make that bathroom safer for my mom. My mom simply did not know that there were measures we could take that would make that bathroom significantly safer for her. We did understand that the engineering and technology and grab bars were available, and we did in fact put a couple of grab bars in the bathtub for her, but we had no idea as to whether those were sufficient, whether they were placed properly, and also, most importantly, whether they would in fact make my mom safe.

As it turned out, our limited efforts, based on limited information, did not make her safe.

The Hunt for Safe Technologies

When I first began conducting interviews for this book, I asked occupational therapists, physical therapists, rehab specialists, visiting nurses, in-home care nurses, orthopedic surgeons—anybody I could talk to!— about bathroom safety, and how we could make bathrooms safer for seniors and those with mobility challenges. Not one of them ever mentioned to me the fact that there are safe bathing technologies, walk-in bathtubs or transition tubs that could be installed to make bathrooms much more accommodating.

It was not until after my mom had passed and my father was facing a double hip replacement that I began to research further.

As I related earlier in the book, my father was told that after the double hip replacement it was possible he would not be able to live independently anymore. The doctor calmly told him that he possibly wouldn't be able to get around without a walker, might not be able to drive, and possibly wouldn't be able to live independently in his home. The doctor matter-of-factly encouraged Dad to plan for those outcomes.

Like many other seniors faced with potential restrictions to their activities of daily living (ADLs), what my father heard was not "possibly," but "definitely"—he was going to be forced into a nursing home. This devastated him, and he called me to defiantly pronounce that he would *never* willingly go into a nursing home. His reaction was based on the fact that he had been traumatized by what had happened to my mom. He had seen firsthand the physical, emotional, and financial toll of her injury and his role as primary caregiver. His quality of life had been terrible. He was helpless to save Mom from her misery in that nursing home, and was adamant that he did not intend to follow her into that situation.

At the same time, he made it equally clear that he had no intention of moving in with either me or my sister. His blunt conclusion: *"I intend to stay in this home. I do not want to move anywhere. When my soul leaves this earth, I want my body to go through that front door, and it is your job, George, to help me make sure that happens!"*

Well, obviously, I got it. It made perfect sense to me that this is what my dad wanted, and it makes perfect sense that I'm going to want the same thing for myself. He lives in the home my mother was born in. He raised his family there. His church is a half a block down the street. His hometown, his friends, his familiar life patterns, his memories—all are right there in that house.

So I busied myself trying to figure out how to keep my dad safe at home. In the process, I began to discover knowledge that I never knew existed. I didn't know about walk-in bathtubs, transition tubs, or safe bathing appliances prior to doing the research in order to help my father out. I didn't know that the bathroom was inherently dangerous and that I could have prevented my mom's injury.

So many of us are in the dark, not aware of the technologies that can enable us to live safely and independently in our own homes for life. This book will provide you with the knowledge and guidance you need to accomplish your objective, just as I did for Dad.

EPIDEMIC #2:   DENIAL
The Waters of Denial Flow Freely

Denial, it ain't no river in Egypt... but it is the leading cause of avoidable deaths and injuries!

I am convinced that one of the primary factors leading to the death and injury of millions of our seniors is a tendency toward denial. Most people that I've talked to—including myself (yes, I am admitting that I talk to myself)—do not openly embrace the issues that we face as we age. If I may say so, it seems to me that men, more so than women, may be inclined to deny our stability, balance, vision, hearing and other age related problems. Being in denial means having no power to do anything about them.

In fact, with my company, Bentley Baths Walk-in Therapy Tubs, we trademarked and use the tagline "Call Before You Fall.®" This tagline came about after two years of helping seniors modify their bathrooms and make them safe and accommodating for them. We displayed our walk-in bathtubs at several trade shows and fairs. I became amused and then frustrated when a senior with advanced mobility issues would hobble up on a walker, barely stable, look at our tub, comment on how wonderful and comfortable it looked, and then deliver the denial kicker: "*Thank goodness I don't need that yet!*" And then they would tootle off on their walkers.

We would look at each other with shock in our eyes and would think—*well if you don't need this safe bathing appliance, then who on earth does?!*

The point is that if we are not willing to be honest with ourselves, and protect ourselves or our loved ones from certain dangers with "pro-aging®" measures, we are going to remain vulnerable to injury.

Our society has sent people to the moon; it is not as though we don't have the capability to manage and cure these illnesses and dangers. I can push a few buttons and talk to my daughter in Thailand without any wires or connections whatsoever, so why would it be impossible to prevent someone from falling? But just as few people know how to build and operate a rocket ship, too few of us know about the huge technological advances that can allow us to age safely. Like my mom and dad said, *"it is impossible to know what we don't know"*. Therefore, we must proactively ask questions, analyze our situations, and commit ourselves to doing something about it.

But, first, we must acknowledge that we are in need of this information. We must admit that we are powerless to stop our aging process, and acknowledge that if we don't take action to protect ourselves…we cannot be protected! That is simply the truth.

On the other hand, once we decide to be honest with ourselves and become proactive to avoid injuries, it is amazing what we can do to improve our longevity and our quality of life.

One of my greatest mentors and role models is Art Linkletter. Mr. Linkletter thrived to the age of 97 and was a very successful, vibrant human being. He wrote and lectured extensively on the issues relative to aging, and I've never forgotten his words to all seniors:

"If you don't feel safe, you are not safe."

We have to self-assess and be honest with ourselves about those activities of daily living which become dangerous as we age. As soon as we experience the first sensation of fear or insecurity, *that* is the time to seek additional information. *That* is the time to ask questions. As my mom said, the only stupid question you can ever have is one that you don't get answered. I hope that this book will stimulate those questions for you.

Let me give you a true example of how denial and ignorance can greatly delay the time we require as a

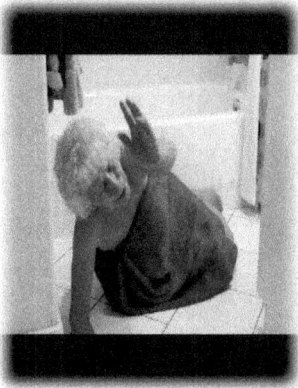

society to embrace and adopt the common use of a new *life saving* technology.

When seatbelts were first introduced, they were not very popular. In fact, I remember my father (and many others) complaining: "Why on earth would I need to wear a belt around my lap just because I'm riding around in my pickup truck? I've never had one before and I've never needed one before."

Well, seatbelts as a safety technology were not developed, promoted and then *mandated by law to be used* just to inconvenience my dad. They were designed to save his life. But we had never experienced this technology before. It was new. There was a lot of misinformation and rhetoric around this new technology when it first came out, and people were prone to cite rationalizations for not using them: "Seat belts will kill me because I'm going to get stuck in the car and I can't get out." "Seatbelts are a death trap, I will burn to death." And the one I really had a hard time understanding (but heard many people express, mostly women): "seatbelts will wrinkle my clothes."

Of course, that was several decades ago. Since then, evidence has been gathered that irrefutably proves that seatbelts save lives. I doubt you know a single person who would *ever* get into an automobile without putting on the seatbelt.

Well, here's my point. Nobody plans to have an automobile accident. But, nowadays, we do put on our seatbelts. Always. Just in case. We always take proactive steps to protect us in the unlikely event we are in a car wreck. It is now *"common sense"* to wear a seat belt. Right?

By analogy, no one plans to fall and injure themselves in their bathroom, and yet everyone ought to take reasonable safety precautions because the dangers are so great.

Let me put this in perspective for you. Let's compare the annual **deaths** caused by all auto accidents with annual bathroom fall-related **deaths** for seniors.

If you truly get the significance of this next fact, you'll call me in the morning. So, think about this...

As of 2009, there were only 30,000 auto accident related fatalities each year counting people _of all ages_. But, there was already a staggering _20,000 fall related fatalities counting only people over 65_!

As stated earlier, the numbers relating to older Americans are going to continue to increase dramatically as Boomers age.

Can it really be true that it is statistically more likely that a senior will die from a bathroom fall than from a car accident?!

And, it is _highly likely_ that each and every one of us will fall and injure ourselves in our bathroom at some point. It is only a matter of time. Have you never slipped, fell, almost fell, stumbled or skidded in a bathroom? Of course you have, but you managed. You can be sure the risk will continue.

Assuming you are younger than 80 and not suffering mobility challenges, how do I help you empathize with what it is like to be over 80 and struggling to use a traditional bathroom? Let me try to help you get a feel for what it is like.

Take the Eighty-Five for Five Challenge

Take five minutes and give a long hard look your bathroom and the way it's configured right now, whether it contains a bathtub or a shower or both. And now, if you are not eighty years old or older, I would like you to imagine that you are. This is a brief experiment to help you better understand what it might be like to deal with your bathroom when you are eighty-five years old. I most certainly hope that you thrive and live vibrant lives to well pass eighty-five years of age.

With that in mind, as you look into your bathroom as it exists now, try squeezing your eyes nearly closed to obscure your vision. Now imagine putting on fifteen-pound ankle weights and a thirty-pound backpack. Spin around as fast as you can five times. Now try to use the bathroom as you normally would.

Here is what you'll experience:

You will not be able to bathe, brush your teeth or have a bowel movement without seriously increased risk. Your balance will be off, your vision will be blurred and you won't be able to stabilize yourself. You will be weaker than you are now. In other words, you will be stressed, and you will struggle! And *you will be at serious risk of falling and injuring yourself.*

You have just experienced interacting with a traditional bathroom as if you were eighty-five years old, or as if you had an illness or injury related mobility issue. There are many, many conditions that we deal with in life that create greater risk of falling. These conditions decrease our stability, our sense of balance and our vision.

Here's another quick thought process. Do you personally deal with any potentially incapacitating disabilities? How many people do you know who are?

If you think not many, think again. Our medical technologies have advanced so far that we often lose sight of just how many debilitating medical conditions we manage as a part of everyday life that would otherwise impair our mobility or quality of life.

For example, do you wear glasses? Maybe just readers? Do you use pain medications, wear hearing aids, or have the benefit of modern dental work? Most people don't think about the fact that without these readily available medical "fixes" we could otherwise be dealing with numerous potentially debilitating conditions that would greatly impact our overall quality of life.

Personally, I would be functionally disabled to a great degree without the convenience of reading glasses. I was just at lunch without my reading glasses, and I literally had to ask someone to read the menu to me. The fact that I can buy them at the drugstore and have them readily available does not mitigate the truth that I would not be able to read without them.

There are many, many people who could not navigate safely in a bathroom without corrective eyewear, or other assistive devices.

The same is true with dental repairs, fillings and other common physical "fixes", without which we would suffer much greater pain and "disability."How many people function with the benefit of hearing aids, knee replacements, pacemakers, etc, etc.

You have just experienced the interaction with a traditional bathroom as if you were eighty-five years old, however, you can go back to your current age or put your glasses back on, or drink cold drinks without pain. Our seniors live with their unique limiting circumstances *all the time.*

Don't just imagine the 85 For Five exercise...DO IT! I insist.

Why? Because...once you do, it will become very obvious that when your bathroom was designed, safety and ease of use with age related conditions were not the primary considerations. You will hopefully immediately realize that you must do something to make your bathroom safer for yourself and your loved ones over sixty-five or who suffer age, weight, injury or illness-related mobility issues.

In other words...don't make them try to read the menu without their glasses! Give them a little help. The technology is here.

You now know it is only a matter of time before you (or they) fall, and hopefully, you will "Call Before You [or They] Fall [®]."

So, you tell me… as with seatbelts, do we really want to continue to make decisions from ignorance or denial when it comes to bathroom safety? Do we really want to require laws and criminal legislation to be passed imposing fines and penalties on all who refuse to make our bathrooms safer? Will we allow *Killer Bathrooms* to continue causing avoidable deaths, injuries and huge costs to individuals and society? Do we really want healthcare costs to skyrocket further out of control before we open our eyes, come out of denial and begin to proactively take action to make our bathrooms safer?

Lord, I certainly hope not. What do you think?

We are at a point in our evolution where we can once again reclaim our control over how we age and the vibrancy with which we live. Are you motivated?

I define "motivation" simply as "motive for action". Can you appreciate how the experience I had with my mother was a compelling motive to take action to prevent the same outcome for my dad? The experience with my dad provided the motive to take action to start Bentley Baths. See a thread here?

Find your "why," and you will take action.

So, the next question I want you to think about is: how do bathrooms get this way and what features are causing the dangers?

CHAPTER TWO

Call Before You Fall®

Safety problems as we naturally age are generally due to the loss of physical capabilities and poor design of bathing equipment. In order to compensate for loss of capabilities, many people tend to over-exert themselves. This seriously affects their security and personal well-being.

For example, older Americans have difficulty bending over and kneeling down. They are unable to access parts of their body when standing, and sometimes even when sitting. Many attempt to challenge their capabilities to access difficult-to- reach areas and injure themselves in the process.

The elderly are constrained by limited reach and poor grip strength. They are required to exert more energy and strength than usual to reach poorly-located water controls. They have problems reaching fixtures and grabbing them. Many receive injuries from applying excessive force.

Poor balance also affects stabilization. This escalates their chances of slipping and falling when entering and exiting the bathtub or shower. So there are many factors that can injure or lead to fall-related injuries.

Unsafe Practices

Both individuals and care providers frequently practice unsafe methods while bathing or assisting with bathing. This is due to not understanding the associated risk level. (I.e., "it is impossible to know what you don't know!") Standing while bathing in the absence of adequate grab bars is the most common of all unsafe practices. Some people stand up to soap their undersides, knowing full well that they have a balance problem. Others reach out to grasp objects, fearing they will fall. Some people store accessories on the bath seat, thereby decreasing the seating area and increasing the chances of sliding off.

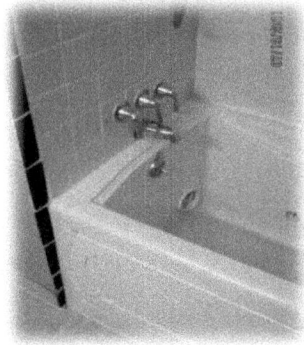

Items in the bathroom are also a big danger. For example, throw rugs or mats outside the tub inevitably lead to tripping and perhaps falling. Objects scattered around the bathroom constitute hazards for everyone, especially those with visual impairments. During the course of my research, I talked to one individual who admitted hanging on to the bathroom door and sink to make transfers — items definitely not designed to bear weight!

A different individual I talked to walks with the help of a walker, but adopted a series of very dangerous methods to make transfers and regulate water temperature. While transferring, he did several complex tasks simultaneously while holding onto the walker with one hand and grasping the wall-mounted grab bar with the other.

He then lifted, dragged and bumped his legs up against the tub. With his hands trembling from the excessive force, he transferred one leg at a time into the tub. The method he adopted for adjusting the water temperature is equally dangerous.

He operated it by kneeling down on the narrow floor space between the tub and the toilet, grasping the walker with one hand and extending himself over the rim of the tub to reach the controls. To complicate things even more, the lighting level in the tub was also very low.

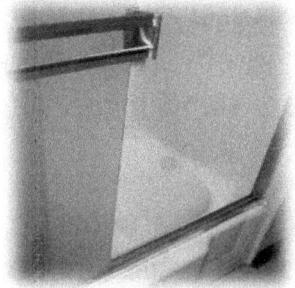

Another person, who had difficulty reaching the controls from outside the tub, regulated the water temperature from the inside and often got scalded. Then there was the daughter who bathed her 90-year old mother in a tub that had no grab bars. The tub was equipped with sliding glass doors.

When stepping in and out of the tub, the mother leaned on the glass doors. Leaning on objects that weren't designed to bear weight will certainly lead to catastrophe sooner or later.

These potential disasters can be permanently eliminated. But first, we must know what they are and take action to eliminate them.

Even though concern for safety is increasing, a large majority of the elderly who live in older homes continue to bathe in unsafe conditions. In spite of all their difficulties, they make no modifications to their outdated bathrooms and expose themselves to unnecessary risk. So I will address each of these in order of the seriousness of the problem.

Survival for less than $100???

Remember my comment earlier about being able to make a bathroom 100x times for as little as $100?

Well, many of the following modifications to *"Eliminate the 7 Killers Lurking in Your Bathroom"* can be completed for very little money, some require no money at all!

#1: Entering and exiting the tub or shower

NOTE: Please visit our Bentley Baths YouTube Channel to view actual videos on seniors going though these processes.www.YouTube.com Keyword: Bentley Baths

You probably already guessed that the number one feature in most American bathrooms that leads to injury is the high sidewalls or thresholds that must be climbed over to bathe. The most common problem is maintaining balance when bathing and making transfers. Those unable to make safe transfers may abandon tub-oriented bathing all together.

Here's what I learned from my research:

Most Americans bathe seven times a week, assuming that there is a bathtub or shower readily available to them. As we begin to experience the stress and difficulty related to bathing, we tend to reduce the number of times that we bathe. Ultimately, seniors are likely to bathe only a couple of times a month, with the average being once per week.

Even that number can be misleading because many of those seniors aren't actually bathing in a bathtub or shower. Many of those are washing themselves by hand in order to avoid transitioning into or out of a bathtub.

Meanwhile, seniors rely heavily on showers, thinking that it's easier to get in and out of a shower. That perceived ease of entry and exit leads to an increase in the number of injuries that occur around the shower. Injuries suffered in a fall entering or exiting from a shower tend to be greater, because the fall is usually from a standing position, and the shower doors and tiled walls and other materials around the shower stall are slick, wet and very hard.

For bathtubs, the issue is not only getting in, but getting up and off the floor after the bath.

Here's an exercise that I frequently conduct with audiences when I am giving a speech: Imagine that you are active and mobile and you begin every day by taking a bath.

You get into the tub, you fill the tub and you do your business. Now it's time to exit the bathtub and go on about your busy day. You pop the drain on the tub and the water begins to leave. Let's start your timer now.

You look around and analyze how to get up out of the tub. You put your hands on either side of the tub and attempt to push your body up off the floor of the tub. But you find out you're not capable of lifting your body up off the floor at this point. This is a troubling new development to you.

So... now you begin to look around and determine how you can leverage yourself up off the floor. You look to the faucet and valves at the far end of the tub beyond your feet. Can't reach and pull without pain. Perhaps the shower curtain will get you up – forget it! Maybe even a soap dish that is near the tub? No way. You begin to test these items to see if they are going to be able to assist you in getting up off the floor of the tub. You struggle, you pull, and you cannot get yourself up. You begin to stress quite a bit and become panicked. You now begin to wonder — *how the h*** am I going to get my body out of this tub?*

Ok, a little shaken, you think to yourself: "Let's get serious here". Now you attempt to roll yourself over. You think that perhaps if you can get on all fours, you might be able to get yourself up and out of the tub. Then it finally sinks in...*no matter how hard you try, <u>you are unable to lift yourself out of the bathtub</u>!* You are stuck.

Now a reality check: At this point, I would guess that you are realistically only *two or even three minutes* into the process of attempting to exit the tub. I have interviewed many people who were stuck in this position—not for two or three minutes, but for hours. In fact, I have spoken to a large number of people who were stuck in their tub for *one, two...and even three days!*

Can you image? Try to imagine the frustration, fear and stress that you would go through being stuck in a bathtub for any extended period of time. Trust me, I can tell you from the people I have interviewed...it is extremely traumatic.

Standing Up is Only Half the Battle

Now let's go through an analysis of exiting the tub once you've gotten yourself to a standing position. From this point, the dangers and risks are now similar for the bathtub and the shower. The only difference, of course, is that you must get your legs up and over the sidewall of the bathtub.

In a standing position, it's very hard to stabilize yourself. There's a very high risk of lightheadedness or a sense of imbalance. When you have wet, slick surfaces like those around a bathtub or shower, you become even more unstable. You may lean on a tile wall; you may place your hand on a shower curtain, a shower hose, a valve or even a towel bar. Towel bars within the bath area are not very common, but they tend to be extremely dangerous when they are located in the shower.

As you start the process of trying to lift your leg and move out of that bathtub or shower, you are at the greatest risk. One slip, one stubbed toe, one loss of traction or slip of a grip and you fall down, onto the hard and unforgiving surfaces of the bathroom.

Statistically speaking, most seniors will experience a fall, or a near-fall, at some point in the bathroom. Once this happens, they become more prone to injury because they are fearful and become overly cautious and tentative in their movements. This is counterintuitive, because it actually increases the instability and loss of security in the transitioning process.

See for yourself, go to our YouTube Video Link: http://www.youtube.com/watch?v=G2C6rzWhAbg

The Bottom Line...

So, having read all this information about how we bathe as we become older... what is the primary method relied on most often by seniors to bathe?

What is your best guess? Is it bathtubs? Showers? What?

Drum roll, please... the most likely answer is...

Neither!

That's right. Neither method is the most frequently relied on method to clean our bodies as we get older and unsafe in bathtubs and showers.

The correct answer is... *sponge baths.*

That's right, it is most likely that the vast majority of seniors in the United States today are reduced to using a *sponge bath* (a/k/a "spit bath" or "French bath") to maintain personal hygiene!

I am sorry, but... how nuts is that!

Fear is Not the Answer

As indicated earlier, a more appropriate response is to make the modifications to the bathroom to increase stability and safety. I interviewed many firefighters and

EMTs while conducting my research. They do far more "lift assists" or "tub pulls" than they do fire calls.

In fact, I was meeting with the fire chief in a small Colorado fire district when he informed me that they do five tub pulls for every fire call.

This really struck me as significant. He jokingly commented that when he first started as a young firefighter 30 years ago, firefighters were known for rescuing kitty cats from trees. Now, that has evolved into rescuing seniors from their bathtubs.

At this point I would like you to think back on the statistics that I gave you earlier in this book. Once every fifteen seconds, a senior in the United States is falling and injuring themselves around their bathroom. How many more fall and require a tub pull or a lift assist and are not accounted for? How many millions more falls happen where the senior does not call the ambulance or the fire department to come help them, and we never hear about it?

When I began to have this conversation with my own father, I was shocked when he finally admitted that he had fallen twelve times in and around his bathroom and never mentioned it to me. Thank God that none of those were serious and he didn't hurt himself (although it is without doubt that he suffered minor overexertion's and strains from each of those incidents). When I queried why he had never mentioned this to me, his only response was "well, I can take care of it myself."

In reality, I now am fairly clear about the fact that my father was afraid that if he informed my sister and me about the frequency of his falls, we would have told him he could not live independently any longer. Therefore, he chose to be silent.

If we are under the age of seven or over the age of 55, it is a fact that we cannot bathe as safely as someone in their twenties, thirties, and forties. It is not that every seven-year-old or every 55-year-old is going to fall every time we try to take a bath, but the fact remains that we are at a higher risk because of our aging process. As healthy as we are, as vibrant as we are, as active as we are, we are still at risk of a fall.

Calling Inspector Gadget

Injuries from falling significantly impact our life expectancy and our quality of life. The smart thing to do is to prevent them from ever happening. Technology solutions are available to resolve the hazards involved in entering and exiting traditional bathtubs and showers.

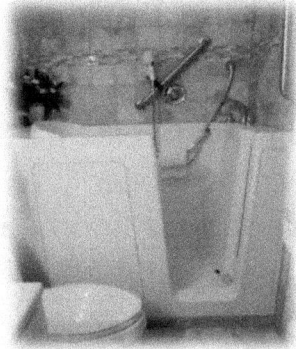

I discovered a technology called walk-in bathtubs during the course of trying to help my father. These tubs are engineered with a high sidewall and a door for entry and exit. A seat is permanently integrated into the bathing well inside the tub.

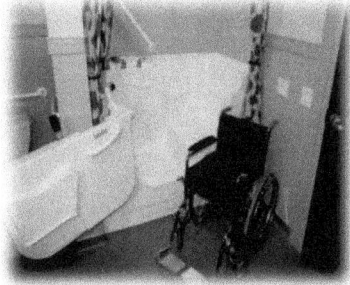

Some of these appliances have outward swinging doors and some of them have inward swinging doors. Either way, one has the ability to enter and exit the tub with a very low threshold. Once seated in the tub, one is perfectly safe. You cannot fall in and you cannot fall out of it.

If the bathtub is appropriately selected based on the bather's body size and mobility issues, it has immense potential to empower all of us to live independently in our own homes for the rest of our lives and *never be forced into a nursing home* because of our inability to bath safely at home. I tell my customers that if you are living in the home you hope to stay in and are over the age of sixty-five, investing in a walk-in bathtub or safe bathing appliance to make your bathroom safer is a *necessity*, not a luxury! It is basically a no-brainer.

There are also transition tubs, a more extreme approach to the bathing appliance. They are designed for individuals with more advanced mobility issues, especially those who rely heavily on walkers, wheelchairs and other assistant devices. Most transition bathtubs are engineered so that the bather can transition directly on to the seat inside the tub and then

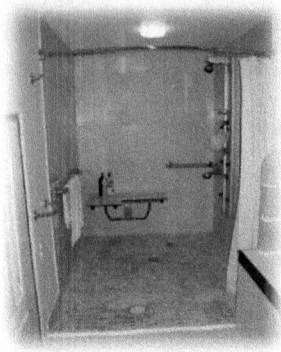

close the door. Again, if properly sized and installed, the bather will be able to enjoy safe, stress-free bathing for the rest of his or her life.

Walk-in or roll-in showers are very commonly relied on as a replacement for traditional bathtubs. While these fixtures may eliminate the danger related to the high threshold in a traditional bathtub, they do not address the safety issues of transitioning into and out of the shower.

However, with appropriate engineering and design, it is possible to fit the shower system with sufficient grab bars and stabilization devices to make it safer. If you acquire a shower system that has an integrated bench, then you will also eliminate the "rain-dance" risks of having to stand and shower throughout the entire bathing process.

That said, I do consider showers to be a poor rest-of-life solution because they eliminate our ability to bathe and soak in a deep soaking environment, and can never provide complete safety and stability. For that, a walk-in or slide-in bathtub is necessary.

The next option in terms of complexity and cost would be processes designed to modify the existing bathroom appliances. I refer to these as Band-Aid responses. A Band-Aid is not a permanent solution, and neither are things like suction-cup grab bars, clamp on grab bars, and moveable grab bars. They are not permanently fixed in the bathing environment. However, there are some mid-level technologies that greatly increase the safety at an only slightly higher cost than the Band-Aids. These mid-level solutions include:

Tub lifts: The most common tub lift used today is basically a chair that sits inside the existing bathtub bathing well and is powered to lift the bather from the floor of the tub up to the height of the sidewall.

This way, the bather can sit on the lift in the higher position and bring their legs over the sidewall of the tub and, if possible, into the tub, and then lower themselves down using the power chair. While this will definitely assist with the "getting up off the floor issue", it does not address the problem of getting ones legs over the threshold and into the tub. Most people I've interviewed are drawn to the idea of a tub lift because they want to try to preserve their ability to soak in a bathtub.

However, because the water in most tubs is only 18 to 22 inches deep, and the tub lift equipment takes up some of that space, it's a serious downside that the bather won't be able to soak comfortably in the tub.

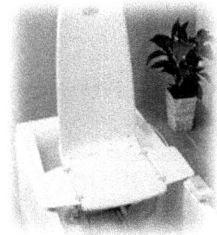

Sling-lift mechanisms: If we are financially required to look at lower-cost solutions and can take advantage of a lift-type mechanism by getting our legs into the tub, I strongly recommend a belt or sling-type system as a lift. This technology uses a sling or fabric band that runs across the width of the bathtub. It is secured and is lowered by an electric motor that allows the bather to lower all the way down to the floor of the tub with only the minimal thickness of the sling material between the bather and the bottom of the tub. I find this far more useful because it permits the bather to experience virtually all of the original soaking depth that they had with their traditional bathtub.

<u>Tub-cuts</u>: Once we determine that we cannot get our legs over the sidewall of the bathtub and into the bathing well, and we cannot afford to do the more appropriate solution of a permanent walk-in bathtub or transition tub, it is possible to consider the process of converting our existing traditional bathtub into a shower. We can accomplish this by cutting out the sidewall of the existing bathtub in order to allow entry and exit as if the bathtub were a shower. It will be easier to get in, but it will be no safer than a regular shower, and we are still facing all the slip-and-fall issues of a regular shower or bathtub.

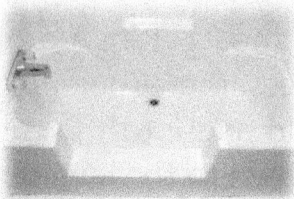

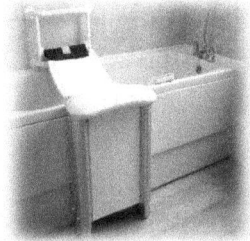

If we combine a tub-cut with a bench or a seat that permanently installed in the tub, then we can have a functional shower with a bench scenario. However, we will not ever be able to soak and bath in this type of setting, and we will also always continue to be less stable.

Tub-cut with a door: One solution is a hybrid between the tub-cut shower option and the chair-lift soak problem. In other words, if I cannot get my legs over the sidewall of the tub, even with a seat to sit on, then I'm going to have to remove the height of the sidewall to be able to get in.

Again, this is the beauty of the engineering behind a walk-in bathtub, as it addresses these issues. If I cut the sidewall of the tub to get my legs in, then there's no reason for me to lower myself through a tub lift or other device because I cannot fill the tub with water. The hybrid tub with a door approach is actually a tub-cut insert, meaning that we remove the material around the sidewall of the tub to allow access.

The insert we install in place of the sidewall actually has a door configured into it. Like a walk-in bathtub, you can step into the tub and close that door behind you, so the bathtub can hold water.

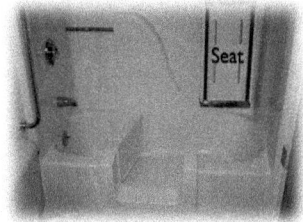

If we combine this with the safety-lift harness system mentioned earlier, we can now enter the tub easily, fill the tub with water, and lower ourselves onto the floor. This "hybrid approach" is the only way that we've determined that would keep the existing bathtub in place and permit the bather to have the safety of entry and exit, and the convenience of being lifted from the floor to the bathtub.

There's no question that the best solution for rest of life is to invest in a walk-in bathtub or transition tub, in order to keep us bathing safely and in our own home for life.

#2: Water Temperature-Related Injuries

The second-worst cause of injuries around the bathtub and shower is unsafe water temperature. This is what is referred to as the phenomenon of "shock and scald." Shock is caused by cold water. Because of the sudden discomfort, the bather instinctively moves quickly to adjust the water temperature or leaves the tub. Scalding is caused by dangerously hot water and can cause burns.

The Americans with Disabilities Act is a really good guideline for these situations. It tells us that we should not be putting water or anything into the bathing environment that exceeds 110 degrees. However, most domestic water heating systems in the United States will store their water between 120 and 160 degrees.

At 110 to 112 degrees, it will take at least twenty-five minutes before that water can cause any skin injury. If we raise that water temperature to 120 degrees, the burn time is decreased to about 19 seconds. Increase the water temperature to 140 degrees and burn time decreases to twelve seconds, and at 150 degrees it's basically less than one second.

But Water Has to Be Hot!

There's a competing problem when it comes to heating water. We should be storing our domestic hot water at higher temperatures than most do. At 120 degrees, we may save a few dollars every year in energy costs, but we actually expose ourselves to higher risk of bacterial infections.

According to the Center for Disease Control, water stored at less than 150 degrees will permit the growth of numerous bacteria that can cause us illness. A number of the colds, flu, runny noses and little illnesses we experience over the course of a year may in fact be caused by bacteria that's allowed to grow in our domestic hot water. We all remember the Legionnaire's Disease event of years ago. This occurrence happened because water was being stored in hotels and on cruise ships below 150 degrees and thus the *Legionella* bacteria was able to thrive in their domestic hot water systems. Many, many people were infected and a large number died. As a result, all cruise ships, hotels and public buildings that serve large populations of people will store their water at 150 degrees, because this is the temperature at which the *Legionella* bacteria cannot survive.

So here are some interesting statistics on hot water:

--131 degrees is the temperature in degrees Fahrenheit that is required to kill the *Legionella* bacteria in a water heater. This temperature must be maintained at all times to keep the water safe.

--Every year in the United States, there are between 3,000 and 4,000 cases of water-related scalds. There is approximately a 30% death rate for those over the age of 60 who experience these scald-related injuries.

--The average water temperature that creates the sensation of pain is 106 degrees. If you factor in the fact that most hot tubs are maintained at 104 to 106 degrees, you can understand why it is so difficult and dangerous for many, especially seniors, to even enter one of these bathing appliances. Pain is felt at 106 degrees, so it is extremely important that our water control processes are effective. It is extremely easy for us to create a situation in which the water entering the bathing environment is hot enough to create pain, resulting in the cycle of shock and scald in order to avoid this painful situation. This is very, very dangerous.

--More than 90% of scalding incidents occur in our home. Young children are particularly at risk because of their tender skin, but the slow reaction time of seniors and those with disabilities make them the most vulnerable to serious hot water burns. Scalding injuries are tremendously painful and the effects can last for years.

Scalding occurs for a variety of reasons. In some cases, water heater thermostats are faulty or set too high, and in others, temperature-regulating valves for the domestic hot water source are either malfunctioning or missing.

How can these problems be resolved? How do we protect ourselves? The answer is the same no matter at what temperature you store your domestic water. We must have sufficient and appropriate temperature control valves installed in all our bathtubs and showers. This is in fact a guideline of the Americans with Disabilities Act.

The issue manifests because we have any number of situations were a bather may accidentally or unknowingly permit water that is too hot or too cold to enter the bathtub. This discomfort makes us move quickly to resolve the problem and therefore exponentially increases our risk of injury. The fact that we are in an individual bathing appliance, and we are not free to move about with ease, increases the risk that our skin will remain in contact with the water long enough to suffer a burn.

Finally, most people shower at a significantly lower water temperature than they bathe. This means our standard approach to plumbing bathtubs and showers in the United States, using a diverter to divert the tub flow to the shower system, sets up a very high risk of injury. If I adjust the water temperature flowing into the tub to what feels to me to be appropriate and I divert that to the shower, I'm at a very high risk of that water being too hot for me, and therefore needing to adjust the temperature to stay in the shower.

If the impact of the scalding water or shocking water does not cause me to fall immediately, I am forced to try to make my way back to the valves to adjust them or turn them off in order to stop the flow. This is extremely unsafe for an 18-year-old, and life-threatening for an 80-year-old. Anything that decreases our focus on being stable and balanced in the bathing environment is a significant factor in increasing our risk of injury.

So what is the answer? According to the Americans with Disabilities Act, every source of water within the bathing environment should have its own anti-scald protection. This means that the tub filler and/or shower should be protected from excessively hot water entering the bathing environment. There are a number of technologies that address this issue, but the bottom line is every single bathtub should be modified to include the installation of an appropriate anti-scald valve.

Most anti-scald valves in the United States are what are called "Type P" thermostatic mixing valves. These are very common in hardware stores and plumbing stores throughout the United States. The "P" refers to the function of a pressure balance between the hot and the cold that is designed into the valve. This is a mechanical process whereby a reduction or increase in the pressure from either the hot or the cold will generate a mechanism to stabilize or balance the pressure between the hot and the cold.

The bottom line for our purposes is that these valves are far better than nothing, but also far from perfect. Pressure balance valves that we commonly use in the United States can have a temperature fluctuation that ranges between five and fifteen degrees, depending on the circumstances.

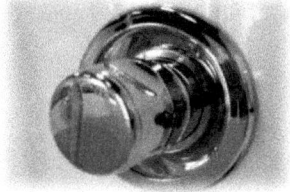

What this means is that if you set the temperature on the valve at a comfortable level and begin the bathing process, if there is a drop in the pressure, the adjustment can create a fluctuation that could range pretty significantly in terms of the water temperature being delivered to the bather.

If someone flushes a toilet, the cold side of the flow to the bath could lose pressure significantly. If the temperature fluctuates significantly, it can still generate uncomfortable and therefore potentially dangerous water temperatures for a senior bather. But again, this technology is far, far superior to no anti-scald valve at all.

By far the best technology is what is referred to as a "Type T" anti-scald valve. These mixing valves are true "thermostatic" valves. That is what the "T" stands for.

A true thermostatic valve physically shuts down the flow of water to the fixture if the mixed temperature exceeds a predetermined level. This approach is the ultimate fail-safe enabling protection within the bathing

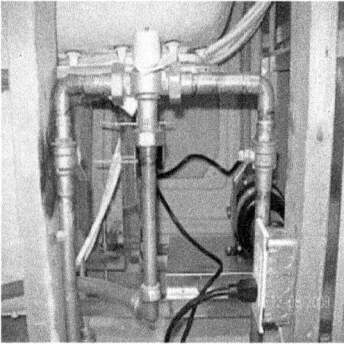

environment. Accordingly, we recommend that every source of water in a bathtub or shower be protected by a true "Type T" thermostatic mixing valve that is sized properly for the appropriate flow.

#3: Poorly-located controls

I honestly never thought about this issue until I started doing the research, and now it seems so obvious to me. As we age, our range of motion, flexibility and grip strength lessen. It becomes difficult to operate faucets, drains and valves safely. Other problems emerge with inadequate reach, poor grasp and low thermal sensitivity. Many individuals indicated to me that because of their inability to bend over and reach low, using controls from the outside of the tub was virtually impossible.

Stretching to reach a valve or drain plug, straining to operate separate hot and cold levers, or maneuvering hard-to-operate controls that require grip strength causes injuries far more often than I had ever realized. Just stand back and look at the average American bathtub. It's five feet long, and the bather is seated at the end opposite the filler valves and drain plugs. *We must be able to reach past our toes to operate the controls!* This is crazy and totally unsafe.

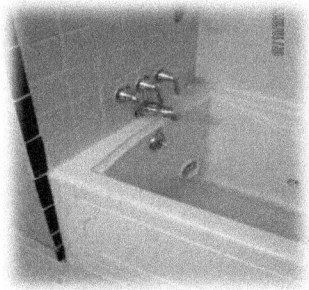

Many American valves will have single control levers that perform multiple functions. As we age, this becomes extremely inappropriate and difficult to deal with. A ball-type control mechanism that must be gripped and twisted to adjust temperature, and levered up or down to control flow, can become virtually impossible to operate with a weak grip.

Now think about the shock and scald of water temperature that can occur under any circumstance. If I've got a valve plumbed into my tub that is difficult to get to and difficult to operate once I get to it, I face a highly increased risk of water related injuries.

The other most frequent control valve in the United States, aside from straight hot and cold flow valves, is a single lever valve that moves the water to full flow immediately. The range of motion of this valve is not to increase or decrease flow, but blends the hot and cold together to adjust the temperature. These valves are very inaccurate and very difficult for seniors to operate in the first instance, and do not protect them from scalding in the second.

Let's look at the design of our bathroom as a clean slate from the perspective of universal design, meaning a design engineered to accommodate us throughout our entire life no matter what health or mobility issues we might develop. This "clean slate" design would involve tub valves and faucets that are conveniently and ergonomically located. I virtually always try to recommend plumbing control valves in the back wall or long wall of the bathing area versus the head wall, wherein most valves are plumbed now. If you can visualize a walk-in bathtub or a deep-soaking appliance with a high sidewall, then flow valves would be situated in the wall directly next to the bather. There would be no reaching or stretching in order to get to a valve.

Next, we would always recommend separating the flow function from the temperature control function. If we can install a high-end thermostatic mixing valve with the flow control or the temperature control lever in the sidewall of the tub surround, the flow valves can be hard plumbed in the wall next to it. This is the very best of solutions for bathers.

Failing this, the next best option is to install the thermostatic mixing valve in the head wall and the flow wall valves at the head of the tub. Keep in mind that with a walk-in bathtub or appropriate safe bathing appliance, those valves are no longer going to be five feet away beyond the bather's feet, but conveniently located in front of them. This is very much like a dashboard in an automobile that is easy to reach.

All valves and control mechanisms should be operated by a lever, and all flow valves should turn to full flow capacity within a quarter-rotation of that lever. Gone forever should be the cross-handled valves of old, where we were required to grip the valve and twist and turn the valve one or more times in order to get a full open flow.

Finally, all lever-operated valves should function with five pounds of pressure or less, and at this level most seniors, even those with very serious arthritis and grip issues or no use of their hands and fingers at all, should be able to safely operate the valve mechanisms.

I'd like to make a note on the topic of showers and showering systems as part of the control of water flow into the bathing environment. Shower systems should flow independently of tub flow systems. This eliminates our reliance on diverters that are most commonly used in American bathrooms. As indicated earlier diverters create more risk of injury because they "hard-divert" the water from the filler system to the showerhead.

When you consider the controls, the wide fluctuation and water temperatures that can flow into our bathtub or shower and the fact that a temperature of 106 degrees is going to create serious pain — combined with the reality that we shower at a significantly different temperature than we bathe — diverting water from the filler spout to the shower is an extremely dangerous activity.

So what's the solution? First of all, we plumb the shower system to flow independently of the tub filler system. This can be done either of two ways. One is through an ADA compliant anti-scald shower valve that is plumbed to a separate handheld shower with the filler system plumbed through its own thermostatic valve.

The other way is for a true thermostatic mixing valve with rapid flow capacity (meaning up to 19 gallons per minute of mixed water) to be installed to flow to both the tub filler system and the shower system. In this case, one flow valve would flow the tub filler, and another would flow the shower. They can be run simultaneously or independently of each other.

I strongly recommend that ADA compliant shower systems with handheld, flow-control-integrated wands be installed in all showers. We should never stand and shower again. Doing the "rain-dance" in a shower stall to get the water on our body where we need it is dangerous.

An appropriately installed handheld shower wand that flows the water and allows us to direct the water where we want it on body makes total sense. The systems that we recommend will actually have a flow shut-off on the wand that gives a senior or mobility-restricted bather much greater control over the flow of the water and allows independent bathing, as well as supporting those circumstances where assisted bathing is necessary. Of course, in both circumstances, we empower the bather to live independently in their own home.

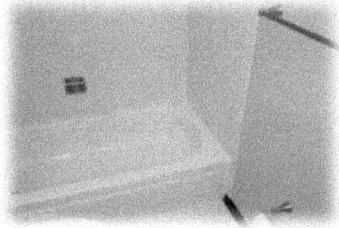

#4: Lack of Support

The bathroom is literally ground zero in the fight against senior-related falls and injuries. As indicated earlier, as many as 80% of all fall-related injuries occur in and around the bathroom. That bathroom has hard, wet and slick surfaces, is very unforgiving, and therefore is exceedingly dangerous. There tends to be no stabilization that is appropriately engineered in most American bathrooms.

Many of the seniors that I've interviewed will literally walk along the furniture, tub, towel bars, or whatever they can lean on in order to support themselves as they navigate through the bathroom. When it comes to transitioning into or out of a bathtub or shower, it can get really ridiculous.

If we are experiencing a lack of stability, especially if we are sensing an impending fall, we are going to grab and reach for anything that we can possibly find to help prevent us from falling. If that item that we reach for is not engineered to support us, it can actually increase the risk of injury.

Towel bars, non-ADA compliant grab bars and grab bars applied by suction can actually create a risk of injury. For example, any bar device, whether it is an adjustable shower, slider, towel bar or grab bar that is greater than 1 ¼ inches in spacing from the wall, can actually set up the risk of a broken arm. With a spacing between the inside edge of the bar and wall greater than 1 ¼ inches, a falling person's hand can slide between the bar and the wall, and as they are falling, they face a very high likelihood of a broken arm or wrist. This happens frequently.

Towel bars and lightweight, adjustable handheld shower or slider bars should be outlawed! *There is absolutely no reason to have a traditional towel bar in a bathroom any more.* These appliances are usually installed horizontally and along the sidewalls at various points throughout the bathroom to hold towels, washcloths and such items.

However, these appliances are installed to the wall with screws and lightweight anchors that are engineered to support the weight of towels, not human bodies that are falling.

A human instinct very similar to fight-or-flight kicks in automatically when we sense great danger. This triggers instantly when we sense we are about to fall. As a result, our mind will instantly look for anything that we can grasp in order to prevent the fall. If I'm in a bathroom, more often than not, what I grasp will not be designed or intended to support me in this process.

A towel bar is very prone to rip from the wall and fail if I grab it as I am falling. Something else also kicks in to increase the risk caused by these towel bars. We have an innate tendency to relax, or take a breath if you will, if we think that the immediate threat has subsided. This happens in a nanosecond. If I think I am falling and I grab a towel bar or some other fixture that is not designed to hold me, there is an instantaneous tendency to relax ever so slightly.

However, if the towel bar or other item fails to support me, I am actually more vulnerable at that point. I'll be even less prepared for a subsequent fall, and be injured even more badly.

It's probably actually better to fall with nothing there than to have a towel bar or something that you grab and it fails. If I am falling, and I know I'm falling, and I have nothing to turn to rely on, I'm actually going to be consciously thinking about preparing myself for that fall all the way down and I have a better chance of controlling my fall, avoiding an item or obstacle that create injury or do a little bit more to protect myself.

Of course, we are talking about very minimal opportunities to avoid injury, but when we are in a life-threatening accident, every little thing that could improve our chances becomes pretty significant.

The solution: *get rid of towel bars*. Get rid of grab bars that are attached by suction. Get rid of inappropriate lightweight grab bars that are not properly anchored in the walls. Replace all of these with ADA compliant grab bars that are properly installed to the studs or with appropriate ADA compliant anchors.

If you have a situation where you are attempting to install a grab bar and you cannot anchor it at both ends on studs or other appropriate mounting material, contact us and we can help you to locate appropriate anchors that will support a grab-bar, even if it is in an open drywall space. In any event, it is important that you have the appropriate stabilization devices for your mobility and safety throughout the bathroom area. You want to be able to navigate through that bathroom, transition into your bathing environment and back out, and be stabilized every step of the way.

#5: Glass Shower Doors and Flimsy Curtains

Let's face it. Hot water, slick surfaces, physical weakness and glass or flexible fabric simply don't go together. The issues around falling into a glass shower door and landing on the sharp edges of a shower door track are significant. When attempting to stand and shower or lower ourselves down or out of a bathtub to soak, the presence of any obstruction, such as shower doors or curtains, greatly increases the lack of visibility and leads to grabbing or leaning on these fixtures for support.

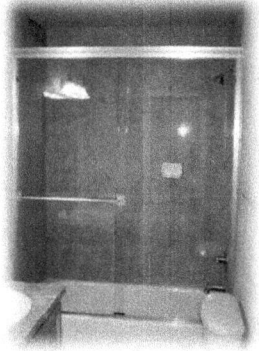

Of course, they are not designed to support a human body and are prone to break or give way, leading to a fall. The presence of glass in a shower door compounds the risk of a cutting injury.

Furthermore, curtain rods and curtain liners create a visual distraction. They also create a risk in the operational process. Anything in the bathroom that distracts the bather from focusing on remaining stable, balanced and safe is a risk factor.

If I am looking up or down trying to fidget with a curtain to get it to shut or open or move out of my way, I am not focusing on my stability.

Curtain rods with rings that stick or do not smoothly slide cause the bather to look up to try and figure out why the curtain rod is not opening up or closing properly, which leads to vertigo, loss of balance, and falling. As with towel bars or anything else, these items are not engineered or designed to support a body. If I have a problem and I feel like I am unstable, I'm prone to grab at the shower curtain or shower door to stabilize myself.

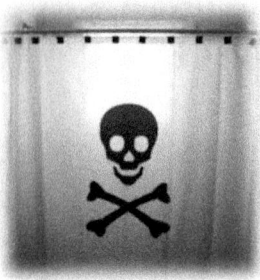

So what's the solution? First of all, if you install a bathing system that is fully ADA compliant and provides you with the water flow and control capabilities discussed previously, there is no need for a shower curtain. No one, no matter their age, should stand up to take a shower.

We want to engineer this bathing environment so we can all sit and be safe during the entire process. A walk-in bathtub or a safe bathing appliance with a high sidewall can be stepped into. We will not be able to fall into or out of such an appliance.

When we sit, showering becomes quite easy. We can reach all of our body parts without any stretching, reaching, strain or risk. We can also use the handheld

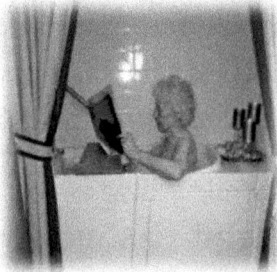

showerheads to easily reach all of our body parts during the showering process. In this way, we can completely eliminate the need for any curtain rods or liners, as well as shower doors.

In the event that we must have some sort of a water barrier or shower curtain in the bathroom, I only recommend utilizing an easy glide track system. If you've ever been in an exam room, in a hospital, or inside of an emergency room, you know that these curtains will easily slide from one end to the other.

Because they are on a track with ball bearings or rollers, the curtains glide smoothly from one end to the other. This will greatly reduce any necessity for tugging, pulling or other distractions from stabilization that could lead to disorientation and falling.

#6 Improper Flooring Material

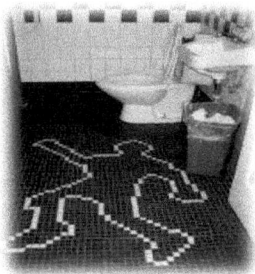

Bathrooms are historically floored with tile or hard, water-resistant surface materials. However, this generally means that these materials offer less traction, particularly in the presence of water. These surfaces become particularly dangerous when we consider factors like; reduced stability due to injury or aging-related conditions, the fatigue and weakness that often follows bathing, or the need for an assistant to help getting into or out of the bath.

Mats and anti-slip pads help, but the risk of feet becoming tangled and tripping on them, as well as the risk of these mats becoming crumpled or moved during use, raises a separate issue of safety.

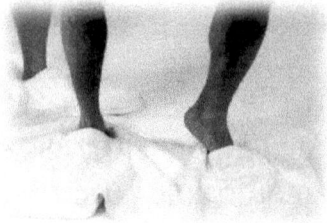

Moreover, mats and pads are rarely a "whole floor" solution. This means there tend to be areas around or away from the mats that are not protected from slipping. Any item that is not securely affixed to the floor can be a hazard. Carpeting in the bathroom helps address the traction problem, but creates issues of mildew, mold and the inability to navigate easily with the use of assistive devices such as walkers or wheelchairs.

The solution: When it comes to flooring, the best solution is a matter of choice, unless you are prepared to invest in some cutting-edge technology. Some modern flooring materials are soft, absorbent *and* waterproof. These tend to be rubberized matting-type materials, or commercial-grade flooring materials with pressure absorbency.

These materials can be installed wall-to-wall in the bathroom, easily accommodate the use of wheelchairs and walkers and, most importantly, provide a cushion in the event of a fall.

The next most likely solution would be a high-gauge sheet floor material that has a cushioned back. Another material that is seeing some successful use is a thicker cork-type material.

Again, these add some measure of cushion, but are not perfect. If tile is going to be used, it is important that each tile be as large in diameter and dimension as possible, and has a significant anti-slip coefficient.

You want the anti-slip function to be fully effective, even in the presence of water on the floor material. Most tile suppliers will have a selection of tile that will meet these guidelines. However, tile is tile, and it is extremely hard and unforgiving to the human body in the event of a fall.

If use of assistive devices is not absolutely necessary, and the bather has the ability to maintain and manage the control of water onto the floor, carpeting definitely provides a safer floor covering in terms of anti-slip qualities and cushion in the event of a fall.

If you are going to use floor mats, it is vitally important that these mats be affixed to the floor in such a way that they will not move, bunch, slip or crumple at any point during bathing process. If any of these factors are capable of occurring, the mats will actually become a dangerous hazard and should be removed immediately.

#7: Lack of Proper Storage and Presence of Clutter

Given that bathroom designs have remained virtually unchanged since the introduction of indoor plumbing, safe accommodation for supplies, towels, and other bathroom related items is grossly inadequate. Many people are forced to place shampoos and bathing soap, brushes, razors and washcloths and other various items

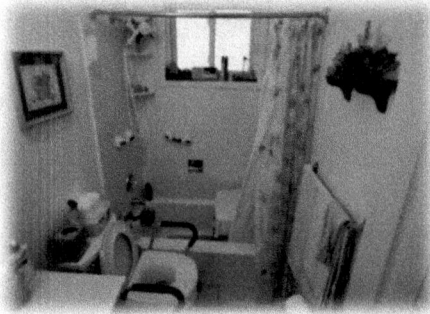

in and around the tub or shower; often in dishes or on add-on accessories in the bathing area. This can lead to accidentally stepping, sitting or leaning on items that result in an injury.

Clutter can also lead to a pain or reflex action (as much with hot or cold or shock or scald issues with water) or slip-related falls. Items on seats, benches or left out about the tub or shower can fall into the floor of the bathing area of tubs and showers, leading to injury or falls resulting from overexertion, over-extension, or loss of stability attempting to retrieve the fallen items.

Many bathrooms lack sufficient storage for towels and other clothing and grooming items. The areas outside the bathing area but in proximity to the bathtub or shower can be cluttered with towels, scales, baskets and the like on the floor, doors and other improper locations. These can lead to tripping or loss of balance while attempting to maneuver around them or trying pick them up for use.

The solution: When installing a walk-in bathtub or appropriate safe bathing appliance, it is important to take into account which items are going to be necessary for the bather to enjoy their baths and have the supplies and items they need. Nothing else should be in the bathroom.

Hampers, clothes, baskets, excess grooming supplies, hair dryers, anything with a cord or table that can be a trip hazard should be removed from the bathroom and located in another spot where the bather can use them safely. The old dressing areas that were common for women prior to the time that we had indoor bathrooms are a perfect example of moving these activities away from the bathroom.

The bather needs open access, what I call a "traffic pattern," from the doorway into the bathroom to the bathing appliance and back out again without any obstacles or hazards in the way.

In the bathtub itself, less is better. Limit accessories, shampoos, soaps and other items in the immediate bath area to only those that are absolutely necessary for that particular bathing experience.

Shelves and support items should be individually located, and suction cupped or adjusted based on the materials within your bathing environment. Just as with your flow valves, think of ergonomics, ease of reach, and lack of exertion to get to any items within the bathtub.

As indicated above, having an item that falls to the floor or is hard to reach can actually set up a significant risk of injury.

Bottom line — be smart and think things through. Minimize anything in the bathroom that is unnecessary and creates clutter. Install the trays, soap dishes and carriers that are appropriate for your specific situation and put items within easy reach while securing them from a fall to the floor.

CHAPTER THREE

YOUR CHOICES MAKE THE DIFFERENCE

FAILURE TO MAKE THE RIGHT MOVES AFTER AN INJURY

After my mom's injury, I watched as my loving, healthy, socially-active father was forced into becoming a primary caregiver. He helped her with all of her activities of daily living. As Mom's condition degenerated rapidly, he also became the primary target of her increasing anger and frustration. Her cognitive abilities decreased significantly due to a series of minor strokes. She became abusive and combative toward him, behavior I never saw from her before.

The stress of dealing with my mother's pain, mental degeneration, and dependence on help actually put him at a very significant risk. I watched helplessly as he, too, deteriorated from all the stress. A major source of stress was caused by his needing to get her into and out of that bathtub to bathe.

Bathing suddenly became an even greater danger! And not just for Mom—_for both of them!_

Following the accident, Mom could no longer bathe independently. We had installed a grab bar on the back wall, and a clamp-on grab bar on the outside edge of the tub.

As Mom was not able to bathe herself any longer, Dad was forced into serving as her bathing assistant. Soon, it was virtually impossible for Dad to bathe her alone in our traditional bathtub. Avoiding slipping and falling on the wet floors was a constant challenge for him, and he was actually over-exerting his back and shoulders trying to lift her and brace her during transitions.

One day, he hurt his back and his rotator cuff trying to transfer Mom into and out of the tub. We were grateful that his injury was minor, but knew that things could NOT continue like that.

He was forced to move her bathing into the shower area so she wouldn't have to step over a sidewall to enter the tub, and also to keep from putting a movable seat inside the tub (we were told to avoid this setup if there was a shower available, as this approach to showering inside the tub was very unstable and dangerous).

We put a waterproof stool and a couple of grab bars into the shower stall, and attached a handheld shower attachment from the old shower spout. I thought we had done the best we could. The healthcare professionals were telling us that this was "all we could do".

No longer being able to bathe was a *big issue* and a major emotional setback for my mom's sense of self-esteem. She *loved* her baths! She loved to soak and enjoy the relaxing escape afforded by spending time in warm water. Access to warm, healthful water was an important quality-of-life factor for her. This turn of events caused Mom greater frustration and stress (and therefore, the same for Dad).

Hiring poorly-trained caregivers to come in proved unreliable and hugely expensive. Plus, my Mother **hated** (and I mean absolutely **HATED!**) the emotional trauma and embarrassment of strangers undressing and bathing her. My mom was always a very private person, and she could not understand why my father would allow for such an indignity. She now had another major point of conflict, stress, and anger with my father.

The simple truth is that my parents' quality of life was at rock bottom for many, many months. Finally, there was no reasonable option (that I knew of) other than a nursing home. Of course, we all told ourselves *"this is only for a while…just until Mom gets better!"* We were completely in denial!

In hindsight, I think we all knew she was never coming back home.

Remember my mom's clearly-stated intention to live in her own home to the end? Well, our being led to believe that we had no choice but to put her in a nursing home was the beginning of the end for my mother. Because of our denial, we did not plan accordingly, and did nothing to change the home to accommodate Mom's potential return. The disappointment, betrayal and sense of failure she felt was visible in her eyes every time we visited, even though she would never say a word about it. She did beg my father to get her out of there. Visiting became a major trauma for them both, but he went every day, twice a day.

Fact is, once in a nursing home, my mom died fairly quickly. Technically, she aspirated, meaning she suffocated on her own fluids. But, I believe my mother decided she had had enough. I believe in my heart that she gave up, and passed away after a few months... to save us all from the financial trauma, and as an acceptance on her part that she would be not be returning home.

My Research Could Have Helped Mom

I have spent the last two years interviewing hundreds of seniors and researching how they treat and manage their pain, illnesses and other health and mobility related problems. I have conducted extensive research into medications and therapies used around the world, and studied objective safety guidelines, such as the Americans with Disabilities Act (ADA) to learn about the treatments and appliances that bring the greatest benefit to suffering seniors.

I learned an amazing truth—using Medical Hydrotherapy® in the home will help treat the core causes of many life-shortening illnesses and painful conditions. Regular use of Medical Hydrotherapy® will greatly enhance digestion, nutrient absorption, skin hydration, detoxification and virtually every aspect of better health for older people!

Water for Life

We all know that water is essential to life. The vast majority of our bodies are water, and over 75% of our brain is composed of water. You may not be a doctor, but you certainly know how to use water as a pain reliever for sore muscles, to treat injuries, ice strains, and as a method of stress reduction. Your own water treatments have been in the form of a hot soak, or a cold shower, and everything in between.

Recently there has been a dramatic swing in medical theory and a long-overdue realization about "healing." The best way to prevent, treat and in many cases cure illness is to give our body the right tools and let it go to work. It is not, as previously thought, to pop pills. Recent studies have confirmed that many of the medications our society has become dependent on, primarily antibiotics and pain relievers, often do more harm than good. For example, antibiotics can be extremely damaging to the liver and have an adverse effect on our natural immune system. The more often we turn to synthetic medicines to overcome infections, the weaker our natural defenses become and the more likely we are to have repeated incidences of infection.

With the regular use of Medical Hydrotherapy®, and the proper intake of healthy water, the right minerals and nutrients our bodies can overcome almost anything.

When it comes to better health and aging safely in place, the best offense truly is a good defense.

What is Medical Hydrotherapy®?

In its simplest form, hydrotherapy can be described as the treatment of illness and injury through the use of water. This includes the use of both hot and cold water, and various methods of use, from soaking to massage. Hydrotherapy treatments help your body get rid of toxins that may be causing joint pain and inflammation, help relax muscles and help relieve pressure on joints and bones. It also relaxes you, both mentally and physically.

Hydrotherapy has been around for thousands of years. Bath houses were the center of social interaction in ancient Rome, and hydrotherapy spas are still popular in Europe, where many were built in large mansions and estates during the 18th and 19th centuries.

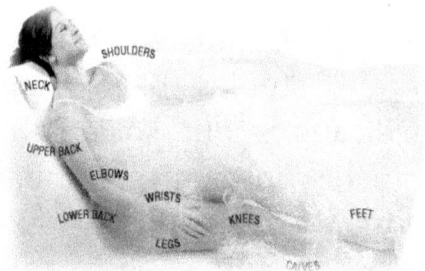

Hydrotherapy is fast becoming a popular and beneficial home health treatment, especially among seniors. It is used to treat common ailments like muscle cramps, muscle weakness, diabetes, circulatory diseases, arthritis, osteoarthritis, back pain, muscle, bone, and connective tissue injuries, balance disorders, and stress and stress-related disorders.

Hydrotherapy makes you healthier in two ways:

1) <u>Thermal Effects</u>: Warm and cold baths alike create certain reactions in your body tissues that help lessen pain and discomfort and improve the healing process. Warm baths open up your capillaries (the small blood vessels in your body that are closest to tissues), which leads to increased blood flow and circulation, helping your body to oxygenate and heal tissue better and get rid of toxins faster. Heat also slows down your internal organs, and is good at lessening certain types of aches and pains.

   Heat increases the production of beneficial body hormones and stimulates the immune system. Warm, moist air from a hot bath can help open up congested or constricted airways in your lungs, throat and sinuses.

2) <u>Mechanical Effects</u>: The gentle tingling, massaging action of air bubbles creates beneficial chemical reactions in your skin and tissues. This leads to increased circulation, which helps oxygenate tissues and evacuate toxins. In water, your body weighs only 10% of its normal weight, so there is a large amount of physical stress removed from your joints and bones, helping to relive pain and discomfort.

   This partial weightlessness also helps relax the

body, because muscles don't have to work as hard to keep the body in position, and are given a chance to relax.

Benefits of Hydrotherapy for Arthritis

One in six Americans has some type of arthritis. It's a fairly common disease that affects our joints, and it usually progresses as we age. Generally, joints swell and become painful and sometimes hard to move, especially after heavy or moderate exertion. As a general rule, the older we get, the more pronounced the symptoms.

Many doctors recommend warm hydrotherapy for treating arthritis. It helps by dilating blood vessels in the body, which in turn relieves pain and eases the tension in nearby muscles, which usually become tense as a result of the pain. It has been shown that warm water treatment is far more effective than dry heat treatments, like heating pads.

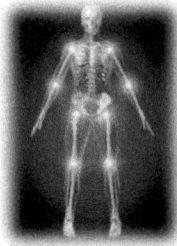

In some instances, doctors will recommend alternating hot and cold treatments, especially for treating the hands and feet. The repeated dilation of the arteries generally has a more profound effect on the reduction of pain in these areas.

Benefits of Hydrotherapy for Lower Back Pain

Behind colds and the flu, back pain is the #2 reason in the United States for doctor visits. Back pain can be caused by a number of things, including stiff or sore muscles, diseases, disorders or injuries of the vertebrae and connective tissue, and pinched nerves. Studies conducted over the last ten years have shown that people who suffer from back pain and who use hydrotherapy as a treatment experience marked reductions in pain versus those people who do not use hydrotherapy. In addition, people who treat their back pain with hydrotherapy use fewer drugs to control their pain, so they don't experience any of the negative side effects associated with some of these drugs.

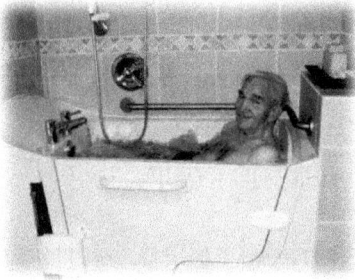

All the thermal and mechanical benefits of hydrotherapy go to work against different types of back pain. Depending on the type of back pain you have, you may experience a substantial decrease in pain, or even a complete eradication of the pain after starting a hydrotherapy regimen. Either way, hydrotherapy makes living with back pain more manageable and provides a relaxing outlet for relief.

Benefits of Hydrotherapy for Insomnia

Almost all people suffer from insomnia — difficulty or an inability to fall asleep — at some point in their lives. For some people, insomnia can be a very severe problem, depriving their bodies of needed rest and making them feel irritable and depressed, and making them more prone to sickness.

Warm baths have been shown to improve both your ability to fall asleep and the quality of your sleep. Hydrotherapy is one of the most popular home remedies for insomnia and sleeplessness.

According to the National Institutes of Health, nerve-signaling chemicals called *neurotransmitters* control whether we are asleep or awake by acting on different groups of nerve cells, or neurons, in the brain.

Research also suggests that a chemical called adenosine builds up in our blood while we are awake and causes drowsiness. This chemical gradually breaks down while we sleep.

Hydrotherapy makes use of water and temperature effects (also called thermal effects) and exploits the body's reaction to hot and cold stimuli. The resulting effect influences the production of stress hormones, invigorates the circulation and digestion, encourages blood flow, and lessens pain sensitivity. Stress, which is a major cause of insomnia, can be easily dealt with through effective use of Medical Hydrotherapy®.

A few hydrotherapy tips to deal with insomnia:

- A warm, soothing foot bath before bed. Fill the tub or foot basin with enough warm water to cover your feet. Add some calming essential oils, sea salt or bubbles.
- Neutral bath has a balancing effect on anxious or irritable people. For neutral bath fill your bathtub with water slightly cooler than body temperature, around 94° F to 97°F (check the temperature of the water with a regular thermometer), and be in the water for some time.
- Take a soothing, relaxing bath. Fill the bath tub with hot water. As the tub fills with water add 2 spoons of Sea Salts to the bath water. Soak for 15-20 minutes. As the water gets cool, replace the bath with warm water.
- Use a blend of oils, herbs and salts while bathing to revive your energy levels and feel relaxed.

Hot baths dilate capillaries in the body and increase blood flow to external areas and to the limbs, drawing blood away from the brain. A lower core body temperature has also been shown to help you achieve a deeper sleep. Soaking in a warm tub at 104 degrees Fahrenheit two hours before bedtime will both lower your core body temperature and draw blood from your brain, priming you for restful sleep. Enjoying the stress-reducing benefits of air jet massages will further relax you and make sleeping even easier.

This Hydrotherapy technique will help you relax and get a natural sleep, so you may not need to take pills.

Benefits of Hydrotherapy for Diabetes

Hydrotherapy has proven useful in helping patients with Type 2 Diabetes. In a study published in 1999 by the *New England Journal of Medicine*, people with Type 2 diabetes soaked in hot tubs for 30 minutes a day, six days a week. Doctors noticed that these patients had an easier time controlling their weight and plasma glucose levels. Some patients even required smaller doses of insulin as a result. Patients who were unable to exercise reported even more benefits, as hydrotherapy helped increase blood flow to their skeletal muscles.

Benefits of Hydrotherapy on the Body

Hydrotherapy is helpful for relieving the symptoms of common ailments found in the torso like chest congestion, bronchitis and asthma. It can also relieve the symptoms of other chest disorders like angina. Soaking the trunk of the body in warm water helps increase blood flow to the heart and lungs and other internal organs, and will help tone muscles, decrease the size of varicose veins, ease nervousness and headaches, and help soothe irritated vocal cords.

In addition, it will help lessen the pain associated with ailments affecting the abdominal and pelvic areas like cramps, hemorrhoids, kidney disorders, intestinal disorders, gall bladder disorders, liver disorders and other systemic problems that cause internal pain.

Arms and legs benefit from increased circulation, especially to the extremities, so cold hands and feet can be alleviated with hydrotherapy. Headaches, migraines, vertigo, rheumatism of the limbs, low blood pressure and nerve disorders of the limbs are also improved with hydrotherapy.

Important Note on Hydrotherapy Treatments

Too much heat or cold can harm you, so it's important that you consult your physician before embarking upon hydrotherapy treatments to be sure the treatment is right for you. Once you and your doctor have agreed upon a treatment, be sure to monitor your progress and report any issues that arise to your doctor. This allows your doctor to make any necessary adjustments to your treatment and protects your health and safety.

CHAPTER FOUR

FINANCES

YOUR HOME IS YOUR CASTLE

Failure to foresee the financial devastation of an illness or injury can be fatal, both physically and financially.

My parents were not wealthy by any means. They had small pensions, some savings and had been relatively financially comfortable. I had put them into a reverse mortgage 15 years earlier, so they had that cash available, and had been able to keep the house up without a mortgage payment.

My mother's accident nearly bankrupted them! Even more sadly, if Mom had not passed away when she did, nursing home and medical expenses would have completely depleted their financial resources.

For example, my parents paid over $30,000 in cash to cover their share of Mother's uninsured medical bills and care requirements stemming from the broken hip and hospital stay. This was nearly half of everything they had in their savings.

This was only the start of their financial devastation. My folks lived in a small community. There are not many in-home caregivers available as resources. Once Dad reached the point where he could not care for Mom, he had to spend thousands of dollars in cash for unreliable, indifferent, low-skilled people to watch Mom. He also had the stress of searching for, interviewing, screening, hiring and firing these people. Not fun!

Please, don't get me wrong. I am not about to fault the in-home caregivers out there. Many are angels! But, like anything else, there are good ones, and there are bad ones. And the *really* good ones are virtually impossible to find. My parents were in a small town, and that further narrowed their options.

When Mother finally went into the nursing home, we thought Medicaid would cover the expense. WRONG! They had failed to plan properly. They learned that Dad had to deplete practically ALL of their savings. Basically, he had to be broke before Medicaid would pick up Mother's nursing home expenses! This also meant Mother could only stay in a nursing home that accepted Medicare/Medicaid—not many did, and those that did were not very high-quality.

My mom's care depleted my parents' savings at a rate of between $5,000 and $10,000 *every single month*.

No one in my family knew what might have prevented the fall in the first place. No one had a clue how to help my dad keep Mom at home, even after the fall. Nor did we know how to help them bathe safely and with dignity, so they could live together in their own home indefinitely. More importantly, not one person in the healthcare community offered any meaningful guidance — before, during or after my mother's injury. Not one doctor, not one physical therapist, nurse, social worker or in-home caregiver ever mentioned any solutions that we didn't know about. We simply had no idea what was possible.

Option One

Do Nothing = INJURY

· **Hospital/ER = $20,000+**

· **Nursing Home = $6k-$12k/mo**

· **Assisted Living = $4k+**

Average Life Expectancy 6-18 mos

75% Never Return Home!!!

Average Cost... $80,000+++!

Don't get me wrong, as with in-home caregivers, there are many well-intentioned, professional caregivers out there who would have helped, had we found them. I am saying that for my parents, in rural Arkansas, no one appeared to help them in a way that would have kept Mom at home.

In hindsight, I *knew*, instinctively, there had to be far superior safety products to the ones we did install for

Mom. There had to be other technologies and resources that could have prevented the fall, or at least kept my mother living safely at home, without putting unreasonable physical, mental and financial stress on my father.

Option Two

Make Home Safe

· Total Home Bath Makeover = $10k-$20k+

· In Home Care = $1k-$12k/mo

· Medical Hydrotherapy = $3k

Average Life Expectancy 5-15 years

75% Never Leave Home!!!

Average Cost... <$20,000!

Over the last seven years, I have avidly sought to help others avoid the tragedy that my family has endured. I felt as though I failed my parents, and I *had* to learn how to help educate my aging father (now 96 years young), to make his home safer and avoid potential falls.

I say I *had* to do this not only because I felt obligated as a son, but also because my dad, like Mom, was adamant that he intended to stay in our family home for *the rest of his life*. How could I ignore his fervent declaration that he would NEVER go into a nursing home? Especially when he had just watched my mom's experience there?

Making my dad's wish come true proved difficult. I needed to learn about products and technologies to make him safe at home. I needed to learn how to create safe and healthy forms of exercise and therapy to enhance Dad's mobility and flexibility.

In pursuing my passion to help Dad, I traveled all over the US, and to Asia, Europe and Canada. I invested thousands of dollars and over 3,500 hours of my personal time researching ALL the products and technologies available.

I actually worked for nearly a year with one of the largest, most highly advertised distributors of walk-in bathtubs in North America. I sat in living rooms and interviewed *hundreds* of seniors, their healthcare providers, and family members in order to determine what issues they faced, and how to best resolve their mobility, health and bathing-related safety issues.

Having invested seven years to extensive research and study, I believe it is fair to say that I am now one of the most experienced legal, safety, health, and "aging in place" consultants working with the elderly and their families in the United States. I am even more confident that I am the leading expert on walk-in bathtubs and safe bathing technologies. I am not saying I know *everything* there is to know. To the contrary... I am saying that I know enough to ask the hard questions that need to be answered to achieve the goal of living independently at home for as long as possible.

I, and all the people in my company, are here to help you in any way we can. But, you need to call us. There are no stupid questions... except the ones you don't ask and get answered.

Call, Before You Fall!

CONCLUSION

Walk-in therapy tubs have the potential to enhance every area of life, provide a safe and sacred environment in which we can not only heal, but flourish and transform adversity into triumph. In short, *THRIVE NOW*. While this may seem a bit dramatic... the truth is... this cannot be denied. Most of us don't have the means or the where-with-all to go down to the neighborhood hot springs for hydrotherapy (assuming there were one). We cannot afford to get the therapies and age appropriate exercise we need without significant hassle and expense.

Many people also do not have access or ability to go to a hot tub. Also, hot tubs, while wonderful for some, need a certain level of mobility, ability to tolerate the heat, and cope with all the chlorine and chemicals that are necessary for most hot tubs. Even a "simple" thing like the loss of self confidence due to illness or injury can have a major impact on a person's mobility.

If you get into a tub, but don't have "confidence" that you're going to be able to get out, what was once a necessary and enjoyable time becomes rife with anxiety and frustration. As I saw interviewing hundreds of seniors and their adult children and caregivers, most seniors "suffer quietly" in their own bathrooms, left to their own imagination as to how to navigate themselves into and out of that tub or shower.

Men in particular are very hesitant to admit they need help, or are not able to safely bath, so they say nothing.

The solution to this is to have your own medical hydrotherapy spa and the appropriate safe bathing appliance for you, installed right in your own home, available to you and your family at any time (day or night) in the safest, most secure and private place there is. That is, your own home.

You can decorate your bathroom however you like. Our surroundings have a profound effect on how we feel about ourselves and how we feel in general. Think about being surrounded in a completely safe, relaxing, rejuvenating environment. Even just *thinking* about that relaxes your mind and body. The brain cannot and does not distinguish between what is *actually* happening and what you *think* is happening.

Notice if you *think* about feeling insecure, unsafe, your body and mind respond by tensing up. You want to live in an environment where everything you want and need will be right at your fingertips… designed especially for you. You have the opportunity with walk-in therapy tubs to bring everything you need right into your own home.

You have before you the technology to turn the ten most dangerous square feet on earth for everyone over 65 (your traditional bathtub or shower) into an "oasis of health and relaxation!"

Right now, right here… we can build the homes of the future. We can be the generation that ends the steady "warehousing" of our elderly and disabled into nursing homes, and all other types of health care facilities. When most people remodel their homes, build a new one or purchase an old one, one of the first things they do is "upgrade" to the latest and best features available. This is done for a variety of reasons, but the top of the list are:

- Adding safety and convenience to their home
- Making their home more beautiful
- Increasing the value of their home
- Preparing for the future
- Wanting to leave their children/grandchildren with the best possible inheritance

Just think about the technological advances in the last ten years: how computers have changed, the constant upgrading of cell phones, iPhones, iPods, tvs, etc. In almost every area of convenience and leisure, technology has steadily advanced. However, in one of the most important, private areas of our lives, our bathrooms, have stayed the same – and bathtubs have remained essentially the same for thousands of years.

The compelling and irrefutable evidence is this: the future is ours if we choose to be among the visionaries and pioneers who make the world a better place for themselves, their loved ones and for people in general. Now is the time to act with intelligence, compassion and integrity.

We have the opportunity right here, right now to be THE generation that moves into this century with the technology of the future blended with the ancient knowledge of the past to provide an environment for healing and hope.

My commitment: Everyone will bathe in a walk-in therapy tub in the future, and everyone will have access to in-home medical hydrotherapy! Join me.

ABOUT GEORGE BENTLEY, J.D.

George is a former law professor and radio talk-show host. He is experienced in the fields of law, business, finance, learning and wellness technologies, personal growth and human development. He has studied at Harvard Law School and New York University School of Law, and is a former Adjunct Professor at the University of Denver College of Law. George is acknowledged as one of the first pioneers in legal Alternative Dispute Resolution, which literally changed the way that law is practiced in this country.

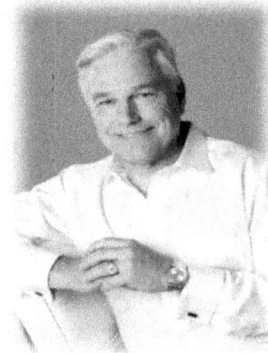

George's mother died in a nursing home from injuries first acquired in a preventable fall at home. Following her death, George committed his life to discovering how to help other seniors avoid the same fate. As an attorney and Certified Aging-in-Place Specialist, George researches accessibility and mobility appliances, cutting-edge health and anti-aging technologies, the Americans with Disabilities Act, and Universal Design Concepts. He writes extensively on safe aging and senior health issues and has personally interviewed and consulted with thousands of seniors, their adult children, and caregivers. He recently finished developing the professional education certifications and coursework for the professional designation of Certified Safe Bathing Specialist, and created the Medical

Hydrotherapy® Program, a unique and revolutionary therapeutic process designed to fight degenerative age-related health problems and help seniors and the health-challenged remain in their own homes. The program has been so well received by the medical profession that virtually every doctor has prescribed it for their patients who desire to enroll.

George is the founder and CEO of Bentley Wellness Technologies, Inc., the nation's leading provider of high-quality, fully Americans with Disabilities Act (ADA) complaint walk-in bathtubs, transition tubs, and safe bathing appliances designed to help seniors live independently in their own homes. He is also the inventor and creator of Medical Hydrotherapy®.

Appendix #1

Safe Bathing Appliance Checklist

DISCOVER CRITICAL <u>FREE</u> INFORMATION YOU NEED TO KNOW <u>BEFORE</u> BUYING A WALK-IN or SLIDE-IN BATHTUB!

All walk-In bathtubs are NOT created equal!

If you do not know the answer to ANY of the following questions, PLEASE CALL US! You also need to know why this information is important. So, if you don't know why a question is on this list: CALL US!

We provide information for all bathers, as well as for current or future assisted bathers. Call us at 800-688-0055 for your FREE *personal and confidential walk-in bathtub evaluation.*

List the make, model and features of EVERY walk-in bathtub you are considering purchasing <u>*before calling for your FREE evaluation!*</u> We will provide you with friendly, professional, objective feedback and help you discover what products will best suit your needs, regardless of the brand you may ultimately decide to choose.

NOTE: All information that _MUST BE KNOWN BEFORE YOU CAN MAKE A BUYING DECISION_ is followed by the toll-free number (800-688-0055). If you do not know this information, it is imperative that you call immediately and we can help you locate that information in order to proceed with the evaluation.

Manufacturer:

_____

_____

Model:

_____

_____

Dealer:

_____

_____

Web Address:

_____

_____

Provide the same information for all models, if considering more than one.

1. Why are you interested in purchasing a walk-in bathing appliance?

- Be specific. Think about your personal issues entering and exiting your current bathing environment, as well as specifics regarding any health or mobility challenges you may be experiencing.

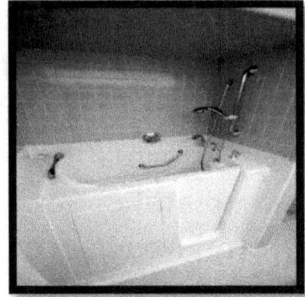

- Is it important for you to be able to live independently for as long as possible in your current home? _____

- Do you want to avoid going into a nursing home or assisted living facility? _____

- Do you require help to exit or enter the bathing environment? _____

- Is bathing/soaking/showering regularly stressful or risky for you? _____

- Would a major injury, hospital stay or nursing home admission impact your financial stability? _____

2. What medical/mobility needs do you have?

- Do you currently use any assistance in your mobility? _____

- If so, is it medical equipment or human assistance?_____

- Which medical health challenges are you currently experiencing?

_____

_____

- Are they expected to worsen over time?

  _____

- Are you currently taking medications? _____

- How many separate prescriptions do you take? _____

- Has anyone told you Medical Hydrotherapy® would be beneficial for you? _____

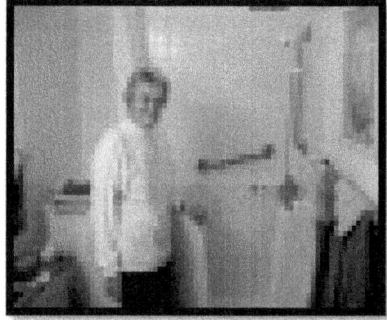

3. Size of Tub

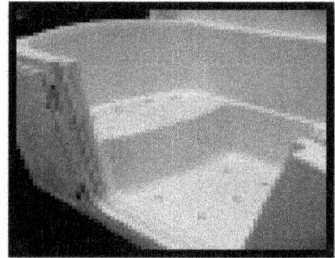

Don't take size of the bathing well inside your bathtub for granted. This is not a "one-size-fits-all" purchase. Making sure the appliance you are investing thousands of dollars to purchase will function comfortably for all bathers is important to your quality of life. Answer the questions below for each walk-in bathtub model under consideration.

- Do you know the overall _bathing well_ dimensions?

  _____

  (NOTE: Not outside tub dimensions, but the inside of the bathing well)

  Dimensions: Height. ____in. x Width____ in. x Length____ in.

- Is this size sufficient for your body shape and size? _____
  (If you don't know, call us at 800-688-0055)

- How many gallons of water does the tub hold? _____ gal.

- What size is your hot water heater? _____ gal.

- Will the water heater provide sufficient hot water to fill the tub? _____

- What is the depth of tub at overflow?_____

- Will the depth of the tub permit mid-chest soaking for all bathers? _____
  (If you don't know, call for help at 800-688-0055)

- Is the seat height ADA compliant and appropriate for your needs? _____
  Do you know the height of seat? _____

- Is this the appropriate height for you? _____
  (If you don't know, call us at 800-688-0055)

- What is the threshold height? _____ in.

- Can you easily clear the threshold height to enter the tub? _____
  (If you don't know, call us at 800-688-0055)

- What are the *outside dimensions* of the tub? (NOTE: These are the dimensions that most manufacturers use to sell their tubs)

Dimensions: Height. _____in., Width_____ in., Length_____ in.

- Are there any issues getting the tub into the desired bathing environment?

  _____

  _____

- How wide is your bathroom door? _____ in.

- How wide is the tub at its narrowest point? _____ in.

- Are there any turns or hallways to pass through to get to the bathroom? _____

4. Safety Devices and Grab Bars

Stabilization location is a very important aspect of making your bathing area safe. You cannot rely on walk-in bathtub manufacturers, dealers, and certainly not salespeople, to provide appropriate devices. If a manufacturer even thinks about stabilization, they tend to treat grab bars as features that are the same for everyone. Nothing could be farther from the truth!

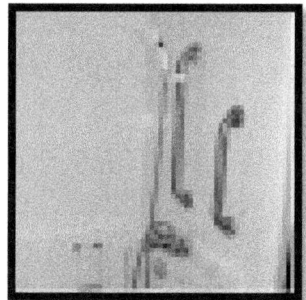

- Does the tub have grab bars built into it? _____

- Are they inside the bathing

area? _____

- Are they located in the correct position for your personal use? _____

- Do they create a hip bruising or other safety issues? _____
(If you don't know, call us at 800-688-0055)

- Are the grab bars and devices ADA compliant? _____

- Will the bars provide appropriate stabilization for every bather throughout the entry and exit process? _____ (If you don't know, call us at 800-688-0055)

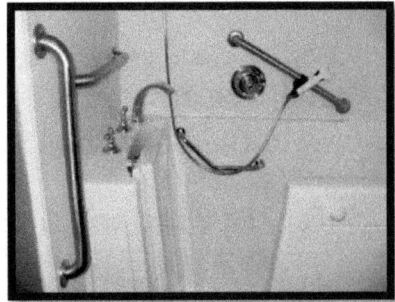

5. Filling and Draining Issues

Walk-in and slide-in bathing appliances create a totally different bathing experience from traditional tubs and showers. You will enter, sit, close the door and wait for the tub to fill. After the bath or hydrotherapy, the bather waits for it to drain before opening the door to exit. How fast the tub fills up and drains is a major quality of life issue for you, and something MOST manufacturers don't even think about.

- What kind of filler valve (faucet) does the tub have?

  _____

  (If you don't know, call us at 800-688-0055)

- Is the flier valve (faucet) independent of the tub, or fabricated into the design of the tub shell? ____

- What size is the filler valve (faucet)? ¾ inch ____ ½ inch _____
  (If you don't know, call us at 800-688-0055)

- Does the tub come with a handheld shower? _____

- How is the shower valve operated?
  Diverter _____ Separately Plumbed _____

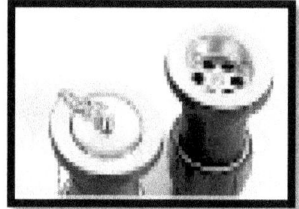

- If separately plumbed, is the shower thermostatically controlled? ____

- Is the handheld shower ADA compliant? _____ (If you don't know, call us at 800-688-0055)

- What is the draining mechanism used?
  Single Mechanical _____
  Single Manual _____
  Single Fast Flow _____

  Dual Fast Flow _____
  (If you don't know, call us at 800-688-0055)

- Is it a sanitary drain? _____
  Cable-operated drain? _____

- Assuming a standard 1½" drain line, do you know how fast the unit will drain? _____ minutes

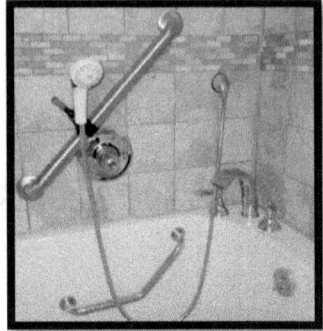

- Does the manufacturer provide a thermostatic mixing valve? _____
What kind of valve is it?
Temperature Protection Valve _____
Manual Blend Valve _____

Pressure Balance Valve _____
(If you don't know, call us at 800-688-0055)

6. Construction Method and Material

There is much confusion in the marketplace as manufacturers tout the benefits of their approach to fabricating walk-in tubs. I do not intend to attempt to go over all aspects of the various construction approaches here. There are only a few bits of information you need to know when it comes to construction-related issues. Remember, a walk-in tub is a "deep bathing well" appliance, and cannot be manufactured as simply or as inexpensively as traditional shallow bathtubs or shower pans. So, how the tub is fabricated is important to long-term satisfaction and performance.

- What is the material used in construction of the

outer skin?
Fiberglass? ___ Acrylic? ___ Both?___
ABS Acrylic?___

- Is the outer surface material non-porous? _____

- Is the manufacturer promoting the use of "leveling legs?" _____

- Does the manufacturer guarantee the shell of the tub? ____

- For how long? _____ years

- Will the manufacturer be able to service the tub locally? _____

- What is the internal structure of the tub?
Metal frame? ___ Integrated wood frame?___
Frameless shell? ___
If metal, is it steel, stainless steel, or aluminum?
_____?

- How are the frame joints connected?
Bolts? ____ Welded? ___ Screws/glue? _____

- How is the shell connected to the frame?
Mechanical connectors? ____
Integrated Frame? _____ Hand laid?____

  Chopped fiberglass? ____

- How is the bathing well supported and integrated to the frame?

Floating frame?___ Plywood flooring?___ Metal joists?___

7. Medical Hydrotherapy®

Without a doubt, one of the most compelling reasons to invest in a walk-in bathtub is the option to add hydrotherapy. We have developed a complete system to this healing technology that establishes a proprietary process we call Medical Hydrotherapy®. However, there are several factors you need to know before deciding what approach is right for you.

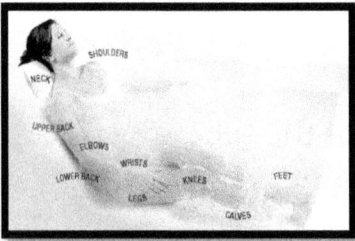

- Is the tub jetted? _____

- Does the manufacturer promote:
Water jetting/Jacuzzi? ___
Air jetting/hydrotherapy? ___
Both? ___

- Which is medically appropriate for you? ___
(If you don't know, call us at 800-688-0055)

- Is the unit self-cleaning? ____

- Are the jets located appropriately for your use? ____
(If you don't know, call us at 800-688-0055)

Now that you have your answers, or maybe even more questions, get together with anyone you want to be involved in the process of deciding, and CALL US at 800-688-0055. We encourage you to have your grown children, spouse, friends or any other trusted advisers involved in this process with you.

Our courteous professionals will walk you and your loved ones through the evaluation of any tub that you have under consideration. We will do the work for you, and help you with the information. Again, we don't care what product you are looking at, or even if you have not looked at all. Either way, our commitment is to help you any way that we can.

We look forward to your call at (800) 688-0055 or e-mail at: Info@BentleyBaths.com.

APPENDIX #2

Whole House Check for Safety
A Home Fall Prevention Checklist for Older Adults

FALLS AT HOME

Falls are often due to hazards that are easy to overlook but easy to fix. This checklist will help you find and fix those hazards in your home.

The checklist asks about hazards found in each room of your home. For each hazard, the checklist tells you how to fix the problem. At the end of the checklist, you'll find other tips for preventing falls.

FLOORS: Look at the floor in each room.

Q: When you walk through a room, do you have to walk around furniture?
Ask someone to move the furniture so your path is clear.

Q: Do you have throw rugs on the floor?
Remove the rugs or use double-sided tape or a non-slip backing so the rugs won't slip.

Q: Are there papers, books, towels, shoes, magazines, boxes, blankets, or other objects on the floor?
Pick up things that are on the floor. Always keep objects off the floor.

Q: Do you have to walk over or around wires or cords (like lamp, telephone, or extension cords)?
Coil or tape cords and wires next to the wall so you can't trip over them. If needed, have an electrician put in another outlet.

STAIRS AND STEPS: Look at the stairs you use both inside and outside your home.

Q: Are there papers, shoes, books, or other objects on the stairs?
Pick up things on the stairs. Always keep objects off stairs.

Q: Are some steps broken or uneven?
Fix loose or uneven steps.

Q: Are you missing a light over the stairway?
Have an electrician put in an overhead light at the top and bottom of the stairs.

Q: Do you have only one light switch for your stairs (only at the top or at the bottom of the stairs)?
Have an electrician put in a light switch at the top and bottom of the stairs. You can get light switches that glow.

Q: Has the stairway light bulb burned out?
Have a friend or family member change the light bulb.

Q: Is the carpet on the steps loose or torn?
Make sure the carpet is firmly attached to every step, or remove the carpet and attach non-slip rubber treads to the stairs.

Q: Are the handrails loose or broken? Is there a handrail on only one side of the stairs?
Fix loose handrails or put in new ones. Make sure handrails are on both sides of the stairs and are as long as the stairs.

KITCHEN: Look at your kitchen and eating area.

Q: Are the things you use often on high shelves?
Move items in your cabinets. Keep things you use often on the lower shelves (about waist level).

Q: Is your step stool unsteady?
If you must use a step stool, get one with a bar to hold on to. Never use a chair as a step stool.

BATHROOMS: Look at all your bathrooms.

Q: Is the tub or shower floor slippery?
Put a non-slip rubber mat or self-stick strips on the floor of the tub or shower.

Q: Do you need some support when you get in and out of the tub or up from the toilet?
Have a carpenter put grab bars inside the tub and next to the toilet.

BEDROOMS: Look at all your bedrooms.

Q: Is the light near the bed hard to reach?
Place a lamp close to the bed where it's easy to reach.

Q: Is the path from your bed to the bathroom dark?
Put in a night-light so you can see where you're walking. Some night-lights go on by themselves after dark.

Other Things You Can Do to Prevent Falls

Exercise regularly. Exercise makes you stronger and improves your balance and coordination.

Have your doctor or pharmacist look at all the medicines you take, even over-the-counter medicines. Some medicines can make you sleepy or dizzy.

Have your vision checked at least once a year by an eye doctor. Poor vision can increase your risk of falling.

Get up slowly after you sit or lie down.

Wear shoes both inside and outside the house. Avoid going barefoot or wearing slippers.

Improve the lighting in your home. Put in brighter light bulbs. Florescent bulbs are bright and cost less to use. It's safest to have uniform lighting in a room. Add lighting to dark areas. Hang lightweight curtains or shades to reduce glare.

Paint a contrasting color on the top edge of all steps so you can see the stairs better. For example, use a light color paint on dark wood.

Other Safety Tips

Keep emergency numbers in large print near each phone.

Put a phone near the floor in case you fall and can't get up.

Think about wearing an alarm device that will bring help in case you fall and can't get up.

How to get up from a fall

1. Prepare

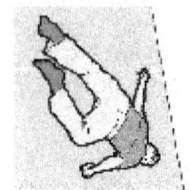

Getting up quickly or the wrong way could make an injury worse. If you are hurt, call for help using a medical alert service or a telephone.

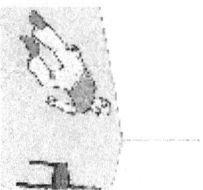

Don't try and stand up on your own.

Look around for a sturdy piece of furniture, or the bottom of a staircase.

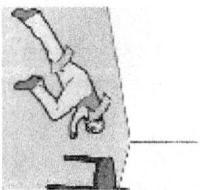

Roll over onto your side by turning your head in the direction you are trying to roll, then move your shoulders, arm, hips, and finally your leg over.

2. Rise

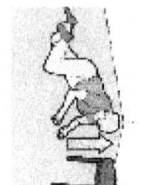

Push your upper body up. Lift your head and pause for a few moments to steady yourself.

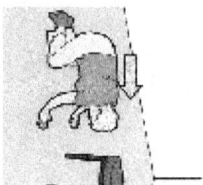

Slowly get up on your hands and knees and crawl to a sturdy chair.

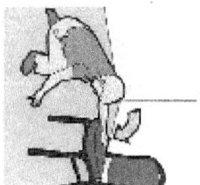

Place your hands on the seat of the chair and slide one foot forward so it is flat on the floor.

3. Sit

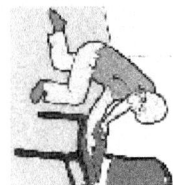

Keep the other leg bent with the knee on the floor.

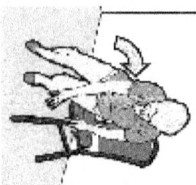

From this kneeling position, slowly rise and turn your body to sit in the chair.

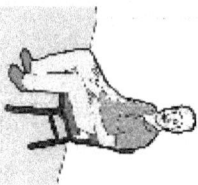

Sit for a few minutes before you try to do anything else.

Talk to your primary care provider about having a fall-risk evaluation. The fact that you have fallen once means you have a high risk of falling again.

KILLER BATHROOM

www.ingramcontent.com/pod-product-compliance
Lightning Source LLC
La Vergne TN
LVHW021510080426
835509LV00018B/2464